International Medical Graduate and the United States Medical Residency Application

Raghav Govindarajan
Sachin M. Bhagavan
Swathi Beladakere Ramaswamy
Editors

International Medical Graduate and the United States Medical Residency Application

A Guide to Achieving Success

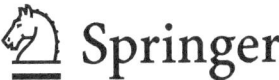 Springer

Editors
Raghav Govindarajan
Department of Neurology
University of Missouri
Columbia, MO, USA

Sachin M. Bhagavan
Department of Neurology
University of Missouri
Columbia, MO, USA

Swathi Beladakere Ramaswamy
Department of Neurology
University of Missouri
Columbia, MO, USA

ISBN 978-3-030-31044-8   ISBN 978-3-030-31045-5   (eBook)
https://doi.org/10.1007/978-3-030-31045-5

This Springer imprint is published by the registered company Springer Nature Switzerland AG
The registered company address is: Gewerbestrasse 11, 6330 Cham, Switzerland

Dedicated to our parents for their constant motivation and support, without which this book would not have been possible!

Preface

Having an opportunity to train in United States is a dream for many medical students from all over the world. And why not? The availability of latest technology along with world-class faculty sets your heart racing. The professional satisfaction you get from practicing here in United States is incredible. At the same time, getting into US residency is not easy, and the competition has been increasing every year. For international medical graduates, it is even more daunting. Candidates from all over the world apply for residency and the number of residency spots has not kept up with the number of applicants which significantly increases competition.

Unlike residency application in many countries where the focus is only on test scores, US residency application is multistep process with test scores being a small component of the entire application. It is this complexity and lack of understanding that makes the application challenging. This journey will test your patience, character and is an expensive process.

To remain focused for this journey, you need adequate information about the various stages of application and means and methods to address them. This book, *International Medical Graduate and the United States Medical Residency Application: A Guide to Achieving Success*, tries to capture the essence of this journey by providing you a glimpse of how your journey should be planned, from writing of USMLE examinations to applying for residency to preparing and acing your interviews.

The book is easy to read, very concise, and crisp, highlighting only what is absolutely important, and has answers to some of the most frequent questions that come during this journey. This is a small effort by the authors and editors who have gone through this long journey themselves and have come out successful and can impart their experiences and shine light on the pitfalls and ways to avoid them for a smooth journey! The book has many tables, figures, and flow charts which makes it easy to read. The book is pocket-sized and can easily fit in your interview jacket or your carry-on bag.

Columbia, MO, USA   Raghav Govindarajan
MD, FAAN, FANA, FACP

Contents

Contributors

Sachin M. Bhagavan, MD Department of Neurology, University of Missouri, Columbia, MO, USA

Tripti R. Chopade, MD B.J. Medical College, Pune, Maharashtra, India

The Wright Center, Scranton, PA, USA

Sorabh Datta, MD Pravara Institute of Medical Sciences, Ahmednagar, India

Lakshmi P. Digala, MBBS, MD University of Missouri, Columbia, MO, USA

Raghav Govindarajan, MD, FAAN, FANA, FACP Department of Neurology, University of Missouri, Columbia, MO, USA

Harleen Kaur, MD Adesh Institute of Medical Sciences and Research, Bathinda, India

Department of Neurology, University of Missouri, Columbia, MO, USA

Nidhi Shankar Kikkeri, MD Drexel University College of Medicine/Hahnemann University Hospital, Philadelphia, PA, USA

Shanan Mahal, MD Southern Medical University, Guangzhou, China

Department of Internal Medicine, University of Arkansas for Medical Sciences-Baptist Health, North Little Rock, AR, USA

Shivaraj Nagalli, MBBS, MD Department of Internal Medicine, Yuma Regional Medical Center, Yuma, AZ, USA

Swathi Beladakere Ramaswamy, MD Department of Neurology, University of Missouri, Columbia, MO, USA

Part I
Pre-interview

Chapter 1
What Does US Residency Application Consist Of?

Swathi Beladakere Ramaswamy

Know your opponent and you will never lose ~Anonymous

US residency is the training you get after your basic medical degree. Candidates who finish their medical school in the US as well as from outside can get into this training. International medical graduate (IMG) is a physician who received a basic medical degree from a medical school located outside of the USA and Canada that is not accredited by a US accrediting body or the Liaison Committee on Medical Education or the American Osteopathic Association. It is the location/accreditation of the medical school and not the citizenship of the physician that determines whether the graduate is an IMG. Thus, individuals who are US citizens when they graduate from an international medical school are US IMGs, and individuals who are not US citizens at the time of medical school graduation are non-US IMGs even if they later become US citizens. Non-US citizens who graduated from medical schools in the USA and Canada are not considered IMGs.

S. B. Ramaswamy (✉)
Department of Neurology, University of Missouri,
Columbia, MO, USA

© Springer Nature Switzerland AG 2020
R. Govindarajan et al. (eds.), *International Medical Graduate and the United States Medical Residency Application*,
https://doi.org/10.1007/978-3-030-31045-5_1

Filling out the residency application (known as MyERAS application) is the last step of the process, but knowing the requirements of application well before you start planning and preparing toward procuring a US residency spot is very crucial. This is because it is this application that actually reflects your achievements, persona and your work toward it. It is this application that paves way to the second part of scrutiny that is interviews. It is a concern that if you don't meet all the requirements within the stipulated time line, it reduces your chance of matching that year and in the coming years as you tend to become older graduate every passing year.

There are certain things that are absolutely necessary before applying, and there are a few things that make the application stand out. A great application is possible with good planning, pure hard work, and clear sense of time line.

List of Various Sections in MyERAS Application

- General Information
- Medical Licensure
- Medical Education
- Medical School Honors/Awards
- Membership in Honorary/Professional Societies
- Experience—Work/Volunteer/Research
- Publications
- Language Fluency
- Hobbies and Interest
- Other Awards/Accomplishments

This application is complete only when it is enclosed with ECFMG certificate (of course! with decent scores), excellent personal statement, curriculum vitae, and three or four personalized letters of recommendation.

Application Tips

- Present the application neatly and free of grammar and spelling errors. All applications should be original.
- Highlight any unique qualifications, academic experiences and volunteer work and test scores on the curriculum vitae.
- Gain experience in a US healthcare facility before applying to a residency to assist in getting a strong letter of recommendation. While letters of recommendation from overseas schools are important, they are not comparable to US schools.
- Ensure the application is filled out correctly, including your NRMP applicant number if you are registered for The Match.
- Write a personal statement that addresses your unique abilities as an applicant.
- Be prepared to answer questions pertaining to your immigration status and visa status if you are a non-US citizen.

Keeping the above requirements in mind efforts to build an outstanding profile that should begin very early in the training; it wouldn't be wrong to say from 1st year of medical school but no later than 3rd year of medical school.

The question as to how to achieve this will be answered in a stepwise manner as you advance through this book

Chapter 2
How Competitive Is US Residency Application?

Swathi Beladakere Ramaswamy and Sachin M. Bhagavan

The best part of competition is that through it we discover what we are capable of, and how much more we can actually do than we ever believed possible ~Anonymous

Over the years, getting into US residency has become more and more competitive. There are various factors that play a role into it. Let's look at various factors that can explain the competitiveness. For our simplicity here, US graduates would mean those who have graduated in US and Canadian schools, and this comprises seniors of US Allopathic School, previous graduates of US Allopathic School, students/graduates of Osteopathic Medical School, and students/graduates of Canadian Medical School. Foreign graduates would mean US IMG and non-US IMG comprising US citizens and non-US

S. B. Ramaswamy (✉) · S. M. Bhagavan
Department of Neurology, University of Missouri,
Columbia, MO, USA

7

citizens who graduated in medical school outside the USA, respectively.

As you can see in Fig. 2.1, there is a steady increase in the number of residency positions every year, but at the same time, the number of US graduates who apply has also increased proportionally. This is because of increase in medical students who graduate in medical school every year which then adds to the applicant pool. While foreign graduates have remained fairly stable and show a slight declining trend because of increasing US graduates, there has been a drastic change in dynamics regarding obtaining appropriate visa for clinical rotation, interviews and residency, and selection of specialty, which further enhances the difficulty for IMGs.

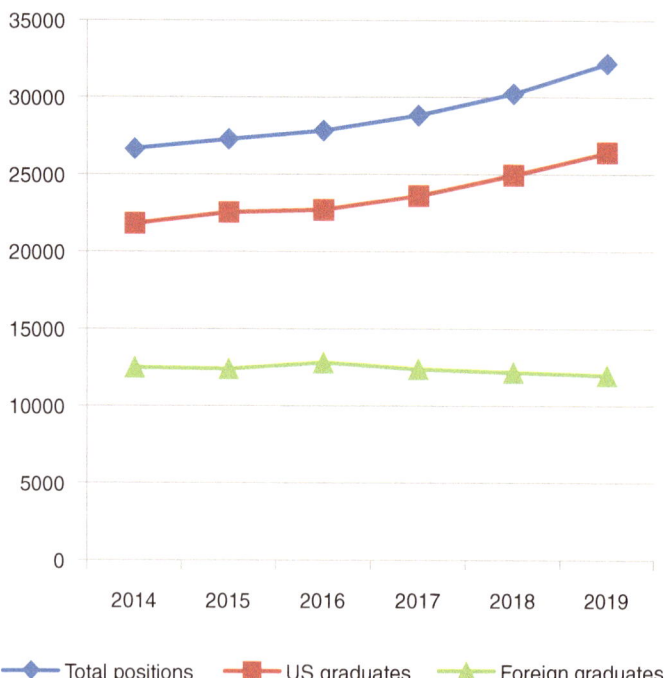

FIGURE 2.1 Trend in number of positions and participation of US and foreign graduates over the years [1]

As shown in Fig. 2.2, match percentage for year 2019, 38,376 candidates participated in match for a total of 32,194 positions. 69% were US graduates, 13% comprised of US IMG, and non-US IMG held a share of 18%.

When it comes to match percentage, US graduates have a fairly stable match percentage of around 94%, i.e., 94% of US graduates every year get matched into residency programs. When it comes to foreign graduates, there has been a steady increase in match percentages for both US and non-US IMG, with 2019 recording the highest match percentage so far with 59% and 58.6%, respectively, as seen in Fig. 2.3. Increase in residency position does play a role, but studies have found that foreign graduates who were successful in matching to their preferred specialty had ranked more programs within their preferred specialty, had higher USMLE steps score, were involved in publication/participation in research projects, and had some experience in the USA (in form of observership or clerkship). US IMG have a slightly higher match rate than non-US IMG. Therefore for having a higher chance of successful match, it is important to emphasize on early planning and building your profile.

One more factor for an IMG to consider before applying is the competitiveness of the specialty and match rates for

Participants in match 2019

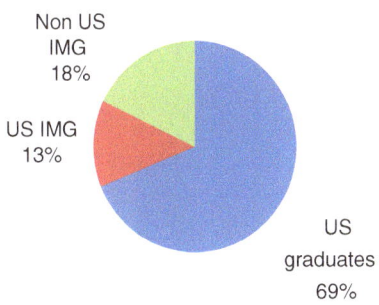

FIGURE 2.2 Percentage of participants from three main categories in 2019

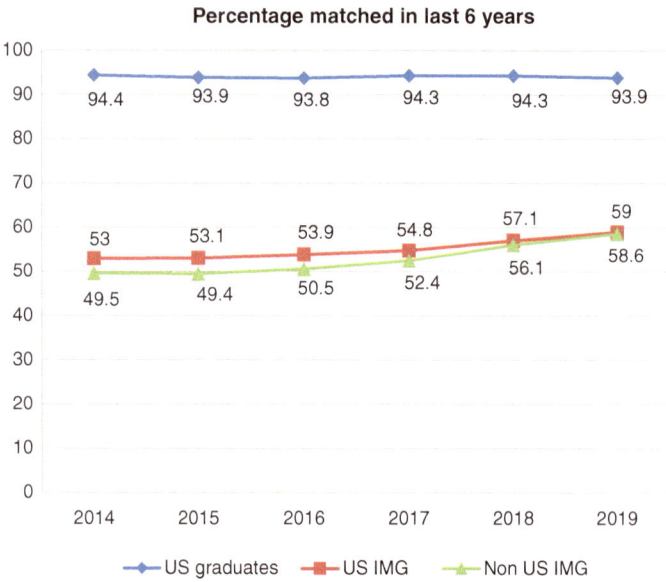

FIGURE 2.3 Trend in match percentage over the years [1]

that specific specialty. There are a few specialties like Internal Medicine and Psychiatry where a lot of IMGs have matched as compared to few specialties like Orthopedics and Plastic Surgery where very few IMGs have matched. Knowing how competitive a specialty can help you narrow down your specialty choices along with the other factors you have in mind such as personal preferences and professional credentials. Having said that, it doesn't mean that you should not apply to those specialties. Competitiveness should not scare you away from specialty you really love. If you are truly passionate about a specialty, you may just have to change your strategy for getting a residency position, put in more work, or take a less direct path. In that case you may have to pad your application with extra work, research, and volunteer experiences and/or complete a preliminary year or transitional year before applying. Once your application is strong, you can further improve your chances by applying to programs that

TABLE 2.1 Showing various specialties categorized based on competitiveness

Less competitive	Medium	High	Extremely competitive
Family Medicine	Anesthesiology	MedPeds	Child Neurology
Internal Medicine	OBGyn	General Surgery	Orthopedic Surgery
Neurology	Physical Med and Rehab	Neurosurgery	Radiation Oncology
Pathology	Diagnostic Radiology	Dermatology	Vascular Surgery
Pediatrics	Transitional Year		Plastic Surgery
Psychiatry			

are best suited for you and applying to enough programs to increase the chance of match. Table 2.1 represents the classification of specialties based on competitiveness according to AAMC data:

Reference

1. NRMP Main Residency Match Data: http://www.nrmp.org/main-residency-match-data/.

Chapter 3
How and When to Get a Clerkship Position?

Swathi Beladakere Ramaswamy

'A negative thinker sees difficulties in every opportunities, a positive thinker sees opportunity in every difficulty' ~Anonymous

Depending on your current stage of medical education, whether still a student or IMG, and your personal medical education career goals, the types of USCE (United States Clinical Experience) available to you vary in benefit. Regardless of which stage you're in, gaining USCE as an international student or IMG is beneficial in the following ways:

1. Acclimating yourself to the US healthcare system
2. Understanding proper procedures
3. Working within the constraints of program protocols
4. Being exposed to clinical staff faculty for mentorship, networking, and more opportunities
5. Learning ACGME programs' core competencies
6. Earning letter of recommendations (LORs) that can eventually strengthen your residency application

S. B. Ramaswamy (✉)
Department of Neurology, University of Missouri,
Columbia, MO, USA

© Springer Nature Switzerland AG 2020   13
R. Govindarajan et al. (eds.), *International Medical Graduate and the United States Medical Residency Application*,
https://doi.org/10.1007/978-3-030-31045-5_3

The ideal duration of USCE is 3–6 months, but more than that is certainly beneficial. It is better if you do it in the department that you aim to do residency in. USCE is two types:

1. Elective/clerkship—Only international students are eligible for this position.
2. Observership—Both international students and graduates are eligible for this position.

Elective/Clerkship is high quality USCE as students get hands on experience and the resultant LOR has more value simply because it is descriptive about student's clinical skills and bedside manners. Electives have an upper hand in impressing a program director (PD) and increasing the chance of being called for interview. Most of these positions can be applied through "FREIDA Online," a webpage that has a list of US programs that offer electives.

How to Apply?

- Go to the Frieda webpage. There are about 150 Medical Schools in this page.
- Find the Universities of your choice. Go to their webpage and select the department of your choice.
- Search for 'Electives/Clerkships'. It will usually be under the 'Education' or the 'Medical Students' section.
- Find out the documents required which will be mentioned in the above page.
- Email the elective/clerkship coordinator that you are interested and re-confirm the documents required to begin the process.

The Usual Documents Required

- Curriculum vitae (CV).
- TOEFL score (English exam).

- Vaccination titers (usually MMR, varicella, hepatitis B).
- Mantoux test/QuantiFERON test (chest X-ray if reactive).
- LORs, about two to three from the faculty of your medical college.
- Personal statement.
- Medical school transcript: It is a document containing a few pages which describe the subjects you have studied in your medical school and the hours of study spent on each subject, duration of postings in each department, consolidated marks card containing scores from all years of medical school, and your general conduct. It can be obtained from your medical school office.
- Step 1 scores (plus/minus Step 2 CK scores). This is the main filtering factor. If you don't have a score, then your options are limited to just five to six places. (They are Harvard, Mt. Sinai, Weil Cornell, Northwestern, Yale, and NIH. Does not mean that they are easy to get either!!)

Some More Things to Know About Electives

- Most electives have application fees ranging from $100 to $500.
- Electives can cost $500 to $2000 per week of rotation! (It is expensive.)
- Some institutes might ask you to get a background check. (Don't panic! You need to just visit some website and answer a few questions. No big deal.)
- Some places might also require you to complete an online Health Insurance Portability and Accountability Act (HIPAA) training. (Again no big deal. Relax!)
- Be in touch with the elective coordinator and humbly ask if you have any questions or concerns (They get hundreds of applications. It's possible that they can forget your existence!)
- If you have anyone you know or from your friends/relatives, in the US medical system, try to contact them and

request them to help you for the opportunity. It helps expedite things and you never know what golden opportunity you might stumble upon. So continue trying to make new contacts and reach out to them.

- Remember, you won't be able to apply for clerkship once you graduate from your medical school. So if you are really interested in doing clerkship, you should plan appropriately.

Visa Requirements

Most places require you to come on F1 (student) visa. Very few places accept B1/B2 (Business/Tourist) visa.

The best time for international students to apply for electives is during their internship year. Apply at least 6–9 months in advance of your desired month of electives to have a much better chance of securing one. Take a break from your internship (3–6 months), complete your US electives during that period, and then return to your medical school to complete the rest of the internship. This would allow you to make the most of the electives and also graduate right in time to apply for residency.

Some private organizations offer clerkships, but these are usually in private clinical setup which most of the time doesn't make a great difference to your application. Choose wisely and these portals are generally opted as a last resort.

Chapter 4
Does an Observership Count?

Swathi Beladakere Ramaswamy

'Opportunities don't happen, you create them' ~Anonymous

The general purpose of an observership is to watch and listen only with no patient contact and no clinical research activity. The observership is undertaken solely for the purposes of gaining knowledge, and there will be no access to clinical systems, no compensation, no fringe benefits, no educational credit, and no employment relationship with the hospital/program in connection with the observership.

In simple words, it involves no hands-on experience, just shadowing another doctor. Most programs do not consider observership as a form of USCE. It's usually done as filler between graduation and residency application. It is fruitful when reasonable time is spent in a big university or community hospital that takes IMGs into residency. Doing observership in a particular region can help getting interviews from that region and it also shows that you are willing to go places without preference. It is true that once you are in USA, it becomes very easy to find more observership spots. There is definitely no harm in contacting program even if you don't

S. B. Ramaswamy (✉)
Department of Neurology, University of Missouri,
Columbia, MO, USA

© Springer Nature Switzerland AG 2020   17
R. Govindarajan et al. (eds.), *International Medical Graduate and the United States Medical Residency Application*,
https://doi.org/10.1007/978-3-030-31045-5_4

meet certain requirements. If the program can't offer a position right now, don't just leave it there. Write a thank you email for their time and request to let you know if spots open in future. Be in touch with the coordinators periodically. The information regarding observerships is usually available on the webpage of respective university/community hospital under medical student/education/observership section. Apply broadly as any opportunity is a good one.

Documents Required

- Curriculum vitae (CV)
- Vaccination titers (some places)
- Mantoux test/QuantiFERON test (chest X-ray if reactive) (some places)
- LORs, about two to three from the faculty of your medical college (some places)
- Personal statement
- Medical school transcript: It is a document containing a few pages which describe the subjects you have studied in your college, duration of postings in each department, your final exam results, and your general conduct. It can be obtained from the college office.
- Step 1 scores (or Step 2 CK scores) (TOEFL scores NOT required)

Additional Information about Observership Application Process

- Many institutes may ask for an observership application fee.
- The observership fee usually depends on the duration (usually 500–1000$/month).
- You have to submit all the documents mentioned before.
- Some institutes might ask you to get a background check and complete online HIPAA training.
- Be in touch with the program coordinator.

Visa Requirements

Most places accept B1/B2 (business/tourist) visa.

Externships

There are observerships which include some hands-on experience. These positions are offered almost exclusively by private agencies or private clinics. The resultant LORs can contain data regarding the hands-on experience obtained. Some programs don't consider this as a form of USCE.

One of the biggest difficulties, you as an IMG might face while looking for observerships is that you might not always get the preferred/applying specialties, and that results in constant dilemma whether it is worth pursuing the different specialty. For example, if you are aiming for observership in medicine but instead you land with Cardiology, Nephrology, Gastroenterology, or Neurology, it is still worth going forward for as these specialties are interlinked. Also, as mentioned before, observership cannot evaluate your clinical skills because you are not in direct contact with patients. Observership gives you a sneak peek into the US healthcare system; in fact, more emphasis is given on your personality like if you are proactive or passive. Are you a team person or are you that kind of person who wants to sail alone? How is your communication skill? Those areas are judged and a letter predominately will speak your personality. However this becomes tricky when the specialty is completely unrelated. For e.g. you are interested in internal medicine but you could manage to get observership in surgery or orthopedics. In those situations, it is not unreasonable to pursue it as you would be wasting your precious time doing nothing instead, but it is always advisable to look around for observership and switch to a more related one when you get. In case you couldn't find one, don't be disheartened; it's not the end of the world. You could still try to work it out by explaining your situation in your personal statement and emphasis on the love of the specialty you are applying. There are a few programs that are very specific about their USCE criteria but majority are not.

According to the NRMP data 2018, there were a few specialties like Emergency Medicine, Diagnostic Radiology, Internal Medicine/Pediatrics, Child Neurology, Dermatology, Orthopedic surgery and plastic surgery, in which matched US IMG have more work experience than who did not match. Across rest other specialties, the average work experiences between matched and unmatched candidates were similar. Non-US IMG had slightly more work experiences than US IMG (5.7 compared to 4.5). At least 85.2% of non-US IMG and 76.9% reported one work experience in US [1]. Therefore it is one of the important aspects of the application. Table 4.1 explains the key differences between Clerkship and Observership.

TABLE 4.1 Comparison between clerkship and observership

Clerkships	Observership
Only students are eligible	Students and graduates are eligible
Responsibilities: Attend rounds, take history, examine patients, present case to the staff, be involved in case discussion/plan/management, type in patient notes	Responsibilities: Attend rounds; observe medical students or residents as they take history and examine patients. Though it is not mandatory, it is beneficial if you involve yourself in case discussions
Most positions are offered by university hospitals	Positions are available in both university and community hospitals
You will obtain hands-on experience	No hands-on experience
More expensive	Less expensive
Very difficult to get into (step 1 score is the filter)	Comparatively easier to get
Prospect of getting interviews from university hospitals increases	The proportion of community hospital interview is more compared to university hospital interviews

Order of Importance

Clerkship> university observership> community externship> community observership> private clinic observership/ externship

Reference

1. NRMP Main Residency Match Data: http://www.nrmp.org/ main-residency-match-data/.

Chapter 5
Does a Research Position Count?

Swathi Beladakere Ramaswamy

Research experience is valuable if it results in publications as at that point it permanently becomes part of your CV. It is less valuable if it does not lead to publications. Compared to any other experience, research work forms the strongest bond with your preceptor/mentor which in an ideal situation leads to one of the strongest letter of recommendation. It is true that research can land you clinical opportunities as well. Most attending (physician/surgeons) do clinical research, and they are aware that as an IMG, your goal is to match into a residency program in the USA. In this setting you can easily and confidently ask them if you can observe them at the clinic. Therefore, the fruitfulness depends on how effectively you are able to obtain benefit from research opportunity.

The additional benefits of research experience are as follows: allow you to better understand published work, determine area of interest, and learn to balance academic and clinical life. The experience also helps you explore and decide about career fields. Many residency programs value research experience, especially academic programs. Limitations of

S. B. Ramaswamy (✉)
Department of Neurology, University of Missouri,
Columbia, MO, USA

© Springer Nature Switzerland AG 2020   23
R. Govindarajan et al. (eds.), *International Medical Graduate and the United States Medical Residency Application*,
https://doi.org/10.1007/978-3-030-31045-5_5

research are that it is time consuming and less rewarding if done for a short period. It is possible to have two to three publications if you dedicate at least 6 months at a big institution with ample ongoing research opportunities and work hard.

Highlights of Research Experience if Done Right

- Adds to research experience and publications/presentations of your CV.
- Gets you a LOR.
- Can pave way to another opportunity of clinical experience such as observership/elective.
- Adds big names to your CV (when done from big institutes/big names).
- An experience that can be elaborated during interviews, helps building a rapport with the interviewer.
- It makes you stand out compared to other applicants, especially if you have publications.
- Helps you make several connections while collaborating with other researchers.
- Demonstrates your interest toward a specific specialty.

According to NRMP 2018, 59.8% reported at least one research experience with an average of 2.1 research experience. 69% of non-US IMGs reported at least one research experience with an average of 2.5 research experiences. There was no specific pattern of the research experience between matches and unmatched candidates across all specialties. However for competitive specialties like Dermatology and General Surgery, non-US IMG who matched had more research experience than those who didn't match.

With respect to some kind of publications, 48.3% US IMG reported at least one publication compared to 65% non-US IMG. The mean publication for US IMG and non-US IMG was 2.9 and 6.2, respectively. There was no specific trend among various specialties; however, in surgical specialties, matched IMGs had more publications than non-matched IMG [1]. Therefore having a research position and/or publication of any kind would help you improve your CV leading to increased match possibilities.

Reference

1. NRMP Main Residency Match Data: http://www.nrmp.org/main-residency-match-data/.

Chapter 6
Do I Need to Do a Master's Program Before Residency?

Harleen Kaur

'Knowledge has a beginning but no end' ~Anonymous

Introduction

A master program is not a requirement for residency application. However, in certain special cases where the applicant wants to apply to a specific specialty branch (Neurology, Surgery, Ophthalmology) such additional courses can benefit the overall application. For older graduates (year of graduation more than 5 years), a master's program can help to improve the application, fill the gap years, and help the applicant to stand out among others. Likewise, a candidate with low USMLE scores can prefer a master's degree or a research program to boost his/her application. Certain foreign medical graduates prefer to take some time off after medical school and join a master's program to gain more experience, for travel and leisure.

H. Kaur (✉)
Adesh Institute of Medical Sciences and Research, Bathinda, India

Department of Neurology, University of Missouri,
Columbia, MO, USA
e-mail: kaurha@health.missouri.edu

© Springer Nature Switzerland AG 2020   27
R. Govindarajan et al. (eds.), *International Medical Graduate and the United States Medical Residency Application*,
https://doi.org/10.1007/978-3-030-31045-5_6

For most fresh medical graduates, planning to apply for residency, do not prefer master degree. Remember, no master's degree can guarantee a residency position; it is an addition to your resume to improve your application and thereby the chances of match in residency.

Type of Master's Program

Master's program may range from short courses to 1-year or 2-year programs. Some applicants prefer online courses as it gives them more opportunity to be flexible with their time. Certain applicants also prefer to have a PhD (Doctor of Philosophy) program before starting their residency. Though master programs can help to improve your academic profile and financial status, these programs are 4 year long and can delay the residency application. Hence the need of a master's program for any applicant depends on his/her own discretion keeping in consideration the gap years, the necessity and its impact on the application.

The most common master's program chosen by applicants includes Masters in Public Health (MPH), Masters in Health Administration (MHA), and PhD in Basic Sciences. Some applicants also prefer short-term courses involving training in specific fields like echocardiography and electroencephalography which again can improve the application.

Benefits of a Master's Program

Getting a master's degree before residency can have several benefits in the residency application:

1. Fill the gap years: Getting a master's degree can be beneficial for older graduates to fill in the gap year and improve their application.
2. Gain academic experience: A master's program is not an additional degree but also improvement in the academic performance and ability to gain better insight into the field of interest.

3. Helpful during the interviews: A master's degree not just improves the application, but can also give content to the interview talks and help the applicants to share their interests with the program directors.

Disadvantages

1. It increases the year of graduation (i.e., the number of years from graduation to residency application): Most programs prefer less YOG and hence might be detrimental to your application.
2. Being away from the medical field decreases your clinical skills which require extra effort to regain them.

Chapter 7
I Am an Experienced International Graduate, Can I Apply?

Tripti R. Chopade

Experience is one thing, you can't get for nothing ~Oscar Wilde

Ashish is an international medical graduate (IMG) who has completed his medical school 5 years back. Later, he completed the internal medicine residency in his home country. At present, he is working as an assistant professor in the department of medicine at an academic institute in India for 2 years. He wishes to move to the United States and wondering whether he can apply for the residency training competing the fresh medical graduates.

Like Ashish, there are many experienced medical graduates from different walks with varying levels of work experiences who wish to know the answer to the question— Can I be successful in getting a residency? Can I apply?

And to answer this precisely, **YES, YOU CAN**!

Experienced IMGs have their unique perks as well as challenges. In this chapter, we will explore in details the realistic possibilities and wonderful opportunities on the path to the residency training for the experienced IMGs, popularly known as 'Old' IMG among the tribe! This

T. R. Chopade (✉)
B.J. Medical College, Pune, Maharashtra, India

The Wright Center, Scranton, PA, USA

© Springer Nature Switzerland AG 2020   31
R. Govindarajan et al. (eds.), *International Medical Graduate and the United States Medical Residency Application*,
https://doi.org/10.1007/978-3-030-31045-5_7

includes anyone who has graduated from medical school five or more years ago. Nonetheless, these experienced IMGs also need to be ECFMG certified before beginning the residency in the United States irrespective of their training overseas [1].

Let's first have a look on the brighter side of being an experienced IMG. The experience may be from prior completion of residency or additional qualifications such as Ph.D., MBA, MHA, MPH, etc. Some might have a substantial contribution to translational or basic science research and might have served in academic practice or have excelled as a clinical educator. The biggest advantage to an experienced physician is a head start during the intern year of the residency training. Once accustomed to electronic health record and hospital system, previously trained IMGs can handle the clinical responsibilities with greater confidence and under minimal supervision. Many programs, especially those with the higher patient load may prefer such experienced graduates.

Remember, all sorts of clinical and academic experiences have shaped you into who you are today and can make you stand apart from the freshly graduated medical school students with yet minimal practical experience. The work ethics honed by such experienced IMGs and the professionalism acquired over the years of patient service can be a great asset during the residency training. One is expected to mature as a physician with time and experiences. An experienced IMG can implement and showcase this maturity by providing the wholesome, empathetic care to patients and a good teammate for colleagues. He can lead the team with a fund of knowledge, creative ideas, and acquired skills. If you decide, you can flip all the odds in your favor.

Being experienced can be a double-edged sword for the residency application. Any sort of clinical experience or skill is seen as added advantage for the residency applicant. However, experiences come with time, and the more time has passed after the medical school graduation, the lesser are the chances for interviews. The bitter fact, many programs automatically filter out the candidates beyond 3–5 years of graduation. Experienced IMGs are facing competition with recent medical school graduates who are perceived to possess the most up-to-date knowledge and more zeal to learn. Being away from a medical school for a substantial period, some may find it difficult to study the basic sciences all over again, and that ultimately affects their USMLE scores. Those in the phase of family settlement may not be able to give their 100% for the match as well as during residency training. Doing the residency training all over again while compromising the privileges of previously earned qualifications is certainly not a cake walk for most of the experienced IMG; it's always better to be realistic, decide the priorities clearly, and then only take the plunge. The entire process of USMLE tests (Steps 1, 2CK, 2 CS, and 3) on average takes 1–2 years and adds additional years along with expenses. Some residency training program faculty members may have the common (mis)belief about the old or experienced IMGs that they are reluctant to learn new things or are less flexible. Some programs might have experienced the arrogance from experienced IMGs that is born out of 'know it all' kind of attitude by being served as physicians for a significant period in their countries. This, of course, varies on a case-by-case basis, and ideally, it's unfair to generalize to all the experienced IMGs. The selection process is largely subjective with very few objective parameters like USMLE scores, and graduation year. The point here is to make the applicants aware of how they are going to be perceived by various interviewers. One must understand the fine line between confidence and arrogance. During shadowing or at an interview, shining out your inner potential in a polite way and keeping an open-minded approach is essential.

Here are some specific suggestions to work on and make your application stand out among the thousands of other applicants while overcoming many challenges.

Setting Clear Goals and Planning

As you embark into the journey of training in the United States, make sure you have well-thought career goals and plans.

I left the well-paid job in my country and decided to start my training all over again to practice in the United States as I wanted to be with my husband who had almost settled here. What I knew about the process of residency matching was just a tip of the iceberg. I was determined to pursue my training, and with the support of my spouse, I was quite perseverant till I got matched after three attempts! It's very important to ascertain whether you really want to do this and make sure to find your own 'why' before diving in this journey. Writing down your career goals, timelines, current financial support, adjustments, and back-up plans if required will help you navigate smoothly.

One of the biggest challenges for experienced IMGS is their year of graduation (YOG). Farther your YOG, more are the chances that your application will be overlooked, especially by the programs which have mentioned clearly about their graduation cut-off on their websites. Many programs prefer the applicants who are within certain years (preferably within 3–5 years) since graduation. Again, this may vary on a case-by-case basis. To make sure your application still gets a fair chance to be thoroughly reviewed by the selection committee and to maximize the chances of being selected for the interviews here are some suggestions based on experiences of those who had been there & some faculty members who have served as interviewers.

Getting Competitive USMLE Scores

Stronger ERAS application opens the door of opportunities for interviews. USMLE scores are one of the significant indicators of your application's strength for most of the programs. If you have not yet taken any of the USMLE steps yet but planning to do so, then read this carefully. First and foremost, aim to get your USMLE scores within a competitive range for the desired specialty. Many programs have a certain score cut-off while filtering the applications. Some residency programs strictly filter the applicants based on number of attempts taken to pass the USMLEs. There is no fixed score cut-off to many programs, and as far as their desired scores, you will be competing with the rest of the applicants' pool. Remember the goal for IMGs is to exceed the credentials of those graduating from US medical schools [2]. Although USMLE scores are not the sole criteria to judge the applicants' eligibility to be a good physician, your impressive scores can certainly fetch you more interviews. USMLE Step1 score reflects your command on basic medical science concepts which is considered to form your solid educational foundation and ability to apply the same in medical practice [3]. Being out of medical school for a significant time and more focused on specialized training afterward, many find it challenging to study the basic sciences all over again. Focus on understanding and revising the concepts in basic sciences, which is a core of the USMLE 1 exam. Step 1 score is the only qualification that is universally available for all applicants during the interview season and prior to the NRMP's ranking deadline [3]. Although, in 2018, the minimum passing score for USMLE Step 1 was 194, the mean USMLE Step 1 score for matched US IMGs was 222.5, and matched non-US IMGs had mean USMLE Step 1 scores of 234.1 [4].

Aim to excel, especially if you are applying for extremely competitive specialties like neurosurgery, dermatology, anesthesia, otolaryngology, radiology, ophthalmology, etc. Take all the USMLE steps seriously and prepare well to get the golden ticket to the residency of your choice. Remember, you cannot change your year of graduation, but your scores are still in your hands. So, work in a timely manner and get the beast under control to make the further journey easier. What if you don't have good scores or have any attempts? —

It's not the ideal situation, but don't get discouraged; there are other ways in which you can still make your application stand out to get in! There are a good number of programs that look for the 'well-rounded' application and won't merely judge you based on scores alone!

Communicating with Programs, Residents, and Co-applicants

Communication is the key to many doors leading you on the path of residency! Connect to previously matched old IMGs; find out the programs which are generous in accepting experienced IMGs. If such programs offer clinical or research experiences, accept those opportunities to create a personalized impact. People love to know the actual person and you get an opportunity to show off your strengths and ascertain that you are beyond your scores. Program coordinators may serve a good source of most up-to-date information regarding the program and learning opportunities as observers/researchers. This certainly helps to wisely apply to the programs where your chances of interviews and matching are more likely. Your enthusiasm to learn & assist with a willingness to shoulder the responsibilities may leave the lasting impression on the program and you may be considered as a potential resident.

Research and Publications

Be prepared and seek the opportunities to present your scholarly work at national and international conferences. Many programs do sponsor the researchers for representing their institutional work at these platforms. Anyhow its long-term investment toward your bright future and all the hard work will pay off once you get residency. As per the latest match data from 2018, most of the IMGs matched in specialties like orthopedic surgery, neurosurgery, plastic surgery, vascular surgery, etc. had a greater number of publications [4]. This highlights the importance of publications if you are willing to be considered for these competitive specialties. The details of how to get the clinical and research experiences, mastering the art of interviews, obtaining personalized letters of recommendation are mentioned in other chapters of this book.

Alternate Pathway

For international board-certified radiologists and orthopedic surgeons there are alternate pathways that allow opting directly for fellowships. It gives an opportunity to practice later as a licensed physician without repeating residency [5]. For further details, the current or former fellows who have pursued this path can be the best resources as well. Ophthalmology and ENT board-certified international physicians can also directly go for fellowships. USMLE steps and ECFMG certificates are must to apply for the fellowships.

Staying Patient and Perseverant

Remember that all the hard work, expenses, and personal sacrifices we make along this path are going to be worthwhile soon when we consistently keep moving in the right direction with full faith in our capabilities. After all, having worked relentlessly in the medical field for a relatively long period, who knows this better than most of the experienced IMGs! Having said this, do not stress out or stretch yourself off the limit. Enjoying the whole process of learning with an open mind is important to avoid the dullness and possible frustration during this journey. You are more likely to rediscover yourselves during this challenging journey**.**

References

1. https://www.ama-assn.org/education/international-medical-education/residency-program-requirements-international-medical.
2. Le T, Bhushan V, Shenvi C. First aid for match (Insider advice from students and residency directors). 5th ed.
3. http://www.nrmp.org/wp-content/uploads/2018/06/Charting-Outcomes-in-the-Match-2018-Seniors.pdf.
4. https://mk0nrmpcikgb8jxyd19h.kinstacdn.com/wp-content/uploads/2018/06/Charting-Outcomes-in-the-Match-2018-IMGs.pdf.
5. https://www.theabr.org/diagnostic-radiology/initial-certification/alternate-pathways and https://www.aaos.org/international/infomedicalgraduates/?ssopc=1.

Chapter 8
How to Prepare for USMLEs, How to Do Well, and When to Take Them?

Lakshmi P. Digala

By failing to prepare, you are preparing to fail ~Benjamin Franklin

What is USMLE?

United States Medical Licensing Examination (USMLE) is a three-step exam for US medical licensure which is sponsored by FSMB (Federation of State Medical Boards) and NBME (National Board of Medical Exam) [1].

- Step 1
- Step 2 – CK Clinical Knowledge
- CS Clinical Skills
- Step 3

International medical students/graduates must apply through ECFMG (Educational Commission for Foreign Medical Graduates) through interactive web application for Step 1 and Step 2 CK and CS. However, Step 3 is applied through FSMB.

L. P. Digala (✉)
University of Missouri, Columbia, MO, USA

© Springer Nature Switzerland AG 2020   39
R. Govindarajan et al. (eds.), *International Medical Graduate and the United States Medical Residency Application*,
https://doi.org/10.1007/978-3-030-31045-5_8

Additional information about the eligibility requirements, the process of applying, fee, scheduling, changes in delivery software, and score report can be obtained from the official website.

Conventionally the American medical graduates start giving their USMLE steps in their M2 or M3 year of medical school. International medical students can start preparing for steps at the same time. It gives an edge over graduates who finished medical school by having the familiarity and freshness of concepts needed, especially for step 1. In this following chapter, we will discuss further how well to prepare and score the best as apart from all the criteria in your application for residency, the key criterion is your score.

Step 1

This test has multiple-choice questions and a 1-day exam divided into 60-minute seven blocks in an 8-hour testing session [2]. The number of questions per block may vary but not exceed total of 280 [2]. It is essential to understand examination format and become familiar with testing software beforehand. Table 8.1 shows the content of the examination with specifications for each category in step 1.

Table 8.2 shows the average distribution of each discipline in Step 1.

Other constructing design for Step 1 and 2 CK is to determine physician tasks and competencies. Percentages may vary to some extent, and updated information will be available in the USMLE website. Table 8.3 shows test-based competency in Step 2ck.

Beyond all the information listed above, the key is to plan your preparation. The key components of your preparation are UWorld self-assessment question bank and Step 1 first aid. Most of the students go for professional coaching like Kaplan, and there are many other tutors out there. However,

TABLE 8.1 The content of the examination with system specifications

System specifications	System range (%)
General principles	13–17
Behavioral health and nervous systems/special senses	9–13
Reproductive and endocrine systems	9–13
Blood and lymphoreticular/immune systems	7–11
Musculoskeletal, skin, and subcutaneous tissue	6–10
Gastrointestinal system	5–9
Biostatistics and epidemiology/population health	5–7
Cardiovascular system	6–10
Multisystem processes and disorders	7–11
Respiratory and renal urinary systems	9–13

TABLE 8.2 Depicts the average distribution of disciplines in Step 1 [2]

Discipline specifications	Discipline range (%)
Pathology	45–52
Physiology	26–34
Pharmacology	16–23
Biochemistry and nutrition	14–24
Microbiology and immunology	15–22
Gross Anatomy and embryology	11–15
Histology and cell biology	9–13
Behavioral sciences	8–12
Genetics	5–9

TABLE 8.3 Shows the test based on competency

Physician tasks/competencies specifications	Competency range (%)
Medical knowledge: applying foundational science concepts	52–62
Patient care: diagnosis	20–30
History/physical exam laboratory/diagnostic studies diagnosis patient care: management	7–12
Health maintenance/disease prevention pharmacotherapy communication/ professionalism	5–7

we stress the fact that first aid, and UWorld are the key parts of your preparation. Make your individualized study plan and practice and make sure you work with UWorld almost every day.

The best time to take this test is when you feel you are ready, which is reflected by your scores in NBME self-assessment. There are many self-assessment exams by NBME that every applicant gives to check where they stand. The score report reflects the final Step 1 score report, and it is your chance to diagnose your weakness if you have any and work on them. These scores are fairly accurate indicators for most candidates of how they would score in the actual exam.

Finally, the test day arrives, and all your hard work is tested by your performance on this big day. In spite of any step examination, below is the checklist that can be of very helpful to improve your endurance and reduce anxiety:

• Make sure you reach the Prometric test center on time or even half an hour early.
• Carry your scheduling permit and ID card (passport/driver's license).
• Given long hours pack your snacks, water, or Gatorade to keep you hydrated.

	Discipline
Discipline specifications	**range (%)**
Medicine	50–60
Surgery	25–30
Pediatrics	20–25
Obstetrics and gynecology	10–20
Psychiatry	10–15

TABLE 8.4 Shows distribution based on subjects. The percentages may vary and would be updated in the website every year [3]

Step 2 CK

It is a 1-day examination divided into eight 60-minute blocks in 9 hours of testing session. This exam focuses on assessing how well you can apply clinical knowledge especially emphasis on health promotion and disease prevention. Table 8.4 shows distribution based on subjects; percentages may vary.

This test key preparation like step 1 includes UWorld self-assessment and first aid. Again, practicing with timed mode prepares you to well acclimatize in managing your time in real exam. There is NBME self-assessment as mentioned above which would be helpful to assess your preparation.

The best time period for IMG students/graduates to give this test is from June to August. It takes 4 weeks to get your score and your transcript becomes available for the match season application.

Step 2 CS

This clinical skills examination tests the ability to gather patient's medical information, performing examination on them and tell them their clinical judgment using standardized patients. It is an eight-hour exam with 12 patient encounters. This exam score output is fail or pass and it is measured as three components described below:

1. CIS — Clinical and Interpersonal Skills
2. SEP — Spoken English Proficiency
3. ICE — Integrated Clinical Encounter

There are only five centers in the entire United States where these exams are conducted. Also, the slots are very limited and they tend to get filled fast. As per USMLE most of the American medical students take in fourth year, and the peak season for this exam is from September to December so you might want to plan to get your preferred test center within time slot [4]. It is always beneficial to keep an eye on the dates 4–6 months prior to taking the test so that you get your desired time frame and centers for the exam. Fig. 8.1 shows the five centers across the United States.

1. Chicago, IL
2. Atlanta, GA
3. Houston, TX
4. Los Angeles, CA
5. Philadelphia, PA

The score report slots are updated in the USMLE website and IMG register and apply through ECFMG on-line services. Being an IMG, this exam is different from the other steps because it tests your communication skills and at the same time efficiency to complete each encounter within

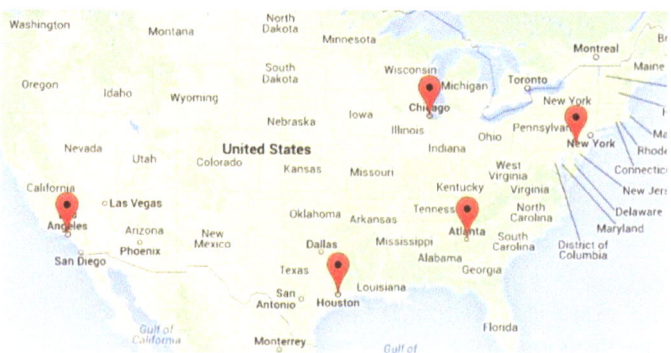

FIGURE 8.1 Shows centers for Step 2CS in US

15 minutes and type the notes in 10 minutes. Therefore, cater more time to practice with friend/family in person to get real experience. We recommend working this with a study partner by setting real timer. Practice to finish the encounter and notes on time. Remember, that in this exam majority of the evaluation is by the standardized patients i.e. the CIS, SEP and some component of ICE. Only a small portion of ICE (clinical notes) is evaluated by a real physician. Therefore it is important to prepare more on how you present yourself to the standardized patients.

Among all the steps, Step 2CS is a challenging exam to many candidates and have frequently seen candidates not clearing this step in their first attempt. Always consider spending extra time in form of more practice/ coaching if you feel you are not confident for the exam. It is not ideal to have repeat attempts on this exam; therefore do not take this exam lightly! It can make/break your application.

Step 3

This is a 2-day exam where on first day, 7 hours of exam is divided into six blocks each; 1 hour of 38–39 questions includes break and tutorial. On second day, total 9 hours exam divide into six blocks of 45 minutes of 30 questions. This day also has tutorial of 7 minutes for CCS (clinical case simulation) where total of 13 cases each were allotted 10 or 20 minutes of real time [5].

Day 1 of step 3 focuses mainly on testing Foundations of Independent Practice (FIP), and on day 2, they test Advanced Clinical Medicine (ACM). On CCS categories showed below are tested.

By now after giving step 1 & 2 all the strategies applied in these two exams is as well applied here. UWorld self-assessment, first aid and NBME self-assessments are again key to prepare well for the exam. Table 8.5 below shows the systems that are tested in the CCS:

Table 8.5 Shows system-wise distribution in Step 3 exam

Immune system
Blood and lymphoreticular system
Behavioral health
Nervous system and special senses
Skin and subcutaneous tissue
Musculoskeletal system
Cardiovascular system
Respiratory system
Gastrointestinal system
Renal and urinary system
Pregnancy, childbirth, and the puerperium
Female reproductive and breast
Male reproductive
Endocrine system
Multisystem processes and disorders

It is not mandatory to give Step 3 for submitting your application for interviews. Most of the American graduates give their Step 3 during their residency years. However, being an IMG, the big advantage of giving Step 3 before match helps getting H1 visa if the program sponsors one. Also, residency would be very busy, and finding time to study and take your exam during that time might become challenging. Therefore, it is always better to take it and get it out of your way. Also, during the selection of interviews or creating a match-list by the programs, among two candidates having a similar profile and scores, taking step 3 could be the difference among two, and you might get added advantage over the other candidate who hasn't taken one. Some programs might require international applicants to finish their step 3. The step 3 results take 6 to 8 weeks to become available, so in order to be ready for applying for a visa, the best time to give step 3 is around January to mid-March. This timeline can be considered hoping to apply for premium processing for H1, which is expensive, but you get approval in 2 weeks.

References

1. https://www.usmle.org/.
2. https://www.usmle.org/pdfs/step-1/content_step1.pdf.
3. https://www.usmle.org/pdfs/step-2-ck/Step2CK_Content.pdf.
4. https://www.kaptest.com/study/usmle/all-about-the-usmle-step-2-cs/.
5. https://www.usmle.org/step-3/#testformat.

Chapter 9
How Can I Make My Residency Application Competitive?

Shanan Mahal

You can't always be the most talented in the room – but you can be the most competitive ~Jamie Shaw

Getting into the residency is a competition. To get a position in residency and that too of your choice, you need to have a strong looking application. In this chapter, we will divide the fields you can work on so that it helps you to build a competitive ERAS application. Fig. 9.1 shows four principal factors that play a role in ERAS application and each of them explained individually as below.

Academic Performance

Getting good USMLE scores of Step 1/Step 2 CK and Step CS, Alpha Omega Alpha membership and Medical Student Performance Evaluation (MSPE).

S. Mahal (✉)
Southern Medical University, Guangzhou, China

Department of Internal Medicine, University of Arkansas for Medical Sciences-Baptist Health, North Little Rock, AR, USA

© Springer Nature Switzerland AG 2020
R. Govindarajan et al. (eds.), *International Medical Graduate and the United States Medical Residency Application*,
https://doi.org/10.1007/978-3-030-31045-5_9

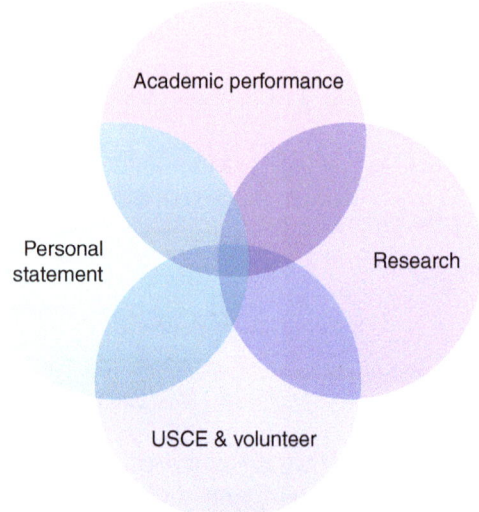

Figure 9.1 Shows four most principal factors which play an important role in your ERAS Residency Application

US Clinical Experience (USCE) and Volunteer Experience

Collecting a strong letter of recommendations (LORs), personalized is more preferred than generic. Try to get it from teaching hospitals or reputable institution as letterhead carries value too. Volunteering in general or related to your specialty reflects your personal interest. Volunteer work also looks good on your CV, for e.g.: you can join American Heart Association (AHA) organization if cardiology is your field of interest, try to participate in Alzheimer or Epilepsy walk if interested in Neurology, if you want to help community put hours in Food Bank.

Research

Having good research experience is important. Try to have a good number of publications, including review articles, and case reports. Participate in a poster presentation and podium presentation in the conferences if possible, e.g., sign up for the American Medical Association (AMA) if you are an Internal Medicine applicant and the American Neurological Association (ANA), if you are a neurology aspirant.

Personal Statement

In this book we have mentioned a detail about how to write your Personal Statement. Your PS reflects your personality. This is the pre-interview that will lend you the interview invite and will help you in ranking as well. Be honest with your PS and follow the chapter given in the book for a good PS.

Tips for making your ERAS application better:

• Use ERAS Tools and materials for learning to make a good ERAS CV and ERAS application.

• Review other people CVs as much as you can. This will help you in shaping your own CV for the application; do not copy them!!

• Your language for the ERAS application and ERAS CV should be simple and easily understandable.

• Try to use active verbs for describing your attributes and your work experiences on the ERAS application. Remember action speaks louder than words.

• Try to name-drop a person with whom you have worked and especially when that person holds good position in the Residency Program where you are applying. That person can vouch for your attributes and work.

• Keep your ERAS application organized. This will reflect your personality.

Chapter 10
How Much Does It Cost to Apply for a US Residency?

Sorabh Datta

> *Do not save what is left after spending, but spend what is left after saving ~Warren Buffet*

Every *IMG* shares that *one* dream. That *one* thing is the *residency*. You have to put too much of your efforts into that dream. Your time, your patience, family sacrifices, those sleepless nights, those moments where you were more concerned for the next day schedule than the present day, that waiting period where you had your fingers crossed for the *USMLE* results, those stationery products which you used during the USMLE preparation, travel expenses, *USMLE* exams fees, etc. All these things surely have some monetary value, but it's not more than the happiness you get when you have achieved your goals. Surely you cannot monetize that happiness. But, yes you can talk about the major expenses that an *IMG* has to bear to apply for a *US* residency, and that is something which you have to be aware of and plan ahead.

S. Datta (✉)
Pravara Institute of Medical Sciences, Ahmednagar, India

© Springer Nature Switzerland AG 2020   53
R. Govindarajan et al. (eds.), *International Medical Graduate and the United States Medical Residency Application*,
https://doi.org/10.1007/978-3-030-31045-5_10

The Cost of Applying for Medical Residency

The cost of applying for medical residency is less as compared to the medical school fees in the United States, but yes it is quite expensive for an IMG. The IMG is mostly not covered by the student loans here in the Unites States, so proper planning is required before applying for the residency programs.

The residency application fees contain two parts:

1. ERAS application fees
2. NRMP fees

The fees depend upon the number of programs applied by the applicant. Table 10.1 shows details about the cost of applying each program.

Payment Methods

Credit card (Visa or MasterCard only) [2].

(Note: Charges will be reflected as "AAMC" on their credit card statement)

TABLE 10.1 Shows more information about the fees based on the number of programs [1]

Number of programs applied	ERAS fees
Up to 10	$99
11–20	$14 each
21–30	$18 each
31 or more	$26 each
USMLE transcript fee	$80 once per application season
NRMP standard registration fee	$85 (up to 20 ranked programs)
NRMP additional programs ranked fee	$30 per program code

Refund Policy

No refund policy by ERAS

Contact Information for ECFMG

- Email: Eras-support@ecfmg.org [3]
- Phone: 215-966-3520
- Website: www.ecfmg.org/eras

Interviewing Cost

There is no specific data available for the average cost an IMG had to bear for applying for the US Residency. As per the AAMC's FIRST (Financial Information, Resources, Services, and Tools) team analysis, the median cost of what an American Medical Graduate (AMG) has to bear for applying for US residency is $3900 with a range of $1000–$7000 [4] (Table 10.2).

For IMGs definitely the price range and the median cost are more. (It could be because of the fact that IMGs apply more programs as compared to AMGs). Figure 10.1 shows three major factors that take up the major cost of the residency application.

- AAMC's FIRST provides financial aid in applying for US residency [5].
- Always plan to cluster interviews, i.e., fly to a region and then travel to all the residency programs of that region through road. This will save expensive air expenses.

TABLE 10.2 Shows average cost for residency application

Median cost	Range
$3900	$1000–$7000
Couples match: $7800	$2000–$15,000

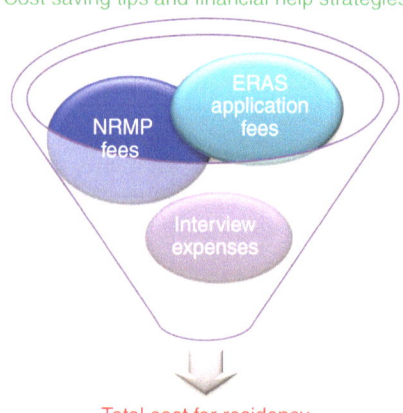

FIGURE 10.1 Shows three major factors contributing for cost

- You can save money by staying at cheap hotels, Airbnb's, places of family or friends, and hostels. (Make sure it is safe!)
- You can cut down your expenses by eating healthy and less expensive foods while traveling.
- If you have done a good research on location you are going to, you can cut down your expenses by using low-cost transportations.
- Try to use hotel's free shuttle service when available.
- If you are going with some friend, you can share your expenses.
- Apply smartly:

  - Research about the programs which are IMG friendly and where your application meets the criteria for their residency.
  - Use services like Fellowship and Residency Electronic Interactive Database (FRIEDA) for narrowing your program search [6].

References

1. The Cost of Applying for Medical Residency. https://students-residents.aamc.org/financial-aid/article/cost-applying-medical-residency/. Accessed 7 Feb 2019.
2. Fees for ERAS Residency Applications. https://students-residents.aamc.org/applying-residency/article/fees-eras-residency-applications/. Accessed 8 Feb 2019.
3. ECFMG|ERAS Support Services. https://www.ecfmg.org/eras/?section=eras&page=index. Accessed 8 Feb 2019.
4. The Cost of Interviewing for Residency. https://students-residents.aamc.org/financial-aid/article/cost-residency-interviews/. Accessed 8 Feb 2019.
5. Financial Aid. https://students-residents.aamc.org/financial-aid/. Accessed 8 Feb 2019.
6. How expensive is it to interview for medical residency?|American Medical Association. https://www.ama-assn.org/residents-students/residency/how-expensive-it-interview-medical-residency. Accessed 8 Feb 2019.

Chapter 11
What Kinds of Visa Do I Need to Apply for and When to Apply?

Nidhi Shankar Kikkeri and Shivaraj Nagalli

Not all who wander are lost ~anonymous

Introduction

A visa is an endorsement on a passport, granted by a country indicating that the holder is allowed to enter, leave, or stay for a specified period of time in a country. A citizen of a foreign country who seeks to enter the United States must first obtain a US Visa, which is placed in the traveler's passport [1]. This chapter highlights the different types of visas available for entry into the US for a non-US resident IMG intending to seek a medical residency. This chapter is by no means exhaustive and be advised that visa rules are constantly changing. We strongly recommend consulting a specialist for visa applications.

N. S. Kikkeri (✉)
Drexel University College of Medicine/Hahnemann University Hospital, Philadelphia, PA, USA

S. Nagalli
Department of Internal Medicine, Yuma Regional Medical Center, Yuma, AZ, USA

© Springer Nature Switzerland AG 2020
R. Govindarajan et al. (eds.), *International Medical Graduate and the United States Medical Residency Application*,
https://doi.org/10.1007/978-3-030-31045-5_11

Why Do I Need a Visa?

A non-US resident international medical graduate would require a visa to visit the United States to give USMLE Step 2 Clinical Skills and USMLE Step 3 exams at designated centers. However, USMLE Step 1 and Step 2 CK can also be given in the United States but not required. The visa is also required for the purpose of doing electives, observerships or externships, research, and attending residency interviews.

What Are the Types of Visas?

The type of visa one must obtain is defined by US immigration law and relates to the purpose of your travel. There are two main categories of US visas:

- Nonimmigrant visas—For travel to the United States on a temporary basis
- Immigrant visas—For travel to live permanently in the United States

We will discuss the nonimmigrant visa options available for an IMG.

B-1 Visa

A B-1 visa is a non-immigrant visa which would allow you to visit the United States temporarily to carry out intended business. Non-immigrant on this visa may not work or participate in patient care and cannot typically stay longer than 6 months since the time of entry to the US.

B-1 visas are available to:

- International medical graduates (IMGs) or students who are coming to the United States to take an elective course at an American medical school or hospital that is part of their formal medical education [2].

• IMGs that come to the United States for observerships or to consult with physicians on the practice of medicine.
• IMGs desirous of coming to the United States to interview for GME positions.

B-2 Visa

The B-2 visa is the visa which allows you to enter the United States with the purpose of tourism, pleasure, or visit to friends and family.

As an IMG, you can apply for either B-1 or B-2 visa to travel to the United States for the purpose of giving USMLE Step 2 Clinical Skills and Step 3 examinations. The usual processing time for B-1 and B-2 visa can vary from a few weeks to a few months. Hence, if your exams are already scheduled on a particular date, it is advisable to apply for these visas early considering the time frame required for the process to complete.

F-1 Visa

F-1 visas are issued to students or researchers who wish to study or conduct research at an accredited US college, university, high school, private elementary school, approved English language school, or other approved academic institutions.

In order to be qualified for an F-1 visa, students must be accepted by a recognized school, college, or university as a full-time student and have proof of sufficient financial support during their stay in the United States. Students issued an F-1 visa are expected to complete their studies within the stipulated time. F-1 visa applicants must obtain an I-20 form from the college or university in order to apply.

Visa Options to Begin Residency

IMGs seeking residency training in the United States usually seek either of the below two visas for residency:

- J-1 visa
- H-1B visa

J-1 Visa (Exchange Visitor's Visa)

A J-1 visa is a non-immigrant exchange visitor's visa which is sponsored by the public or private entities approved by the US Department of State for the purpose of teaching, instructing or lecturing, studying, observing, conducting research, consulting, demonstrating special skills, or receiving training or graduate medical education or training.

ECFMG (Educational Commission for Foreign Medical Graduates) is authorized by the US Department of State to sponsor J-1 Exchange Visitor physicians enrolled in accredited programs of graduate medical education or training or advanced research programs. Many universities and research institutions in the United States are authorized to sponsor Exchange Visitors in the categories of student or research scholar [3].

The J-1 visa is a temporary nonimmigrant visa reserved for participants in the Exchange Visitor Program and can be used for graduate medical education and training. It is valid for a maximum period of 7 years.

Currently, this is the most common visa accepted by the residency programs to begin the residency.

Upon completion of J-1 stay in the US, you will be required to return to your home country for a period of at least 2 years. This requirement can be waived by serving in a medically underserved area in the United States for a period of 3 years (J-1 waiver program).

Another lesser known fact is that families of J-1, who will be given J-2 visa, are eligible to work [4]. However, they need to apply and secure Employment authorization document (EAD) after proper submission of documents to the United States Citizenship and Immigration Services (USCIS).

H-1B Visa

An H-1B visa is another temporary non-immigrant visa where you are authorized to work. The H-1B visa program allows companies in the United States to temporarily employ foreign workers in the occupations that require the theoretical and practical application of a body of highly specialized knowledge and a bachelor's degree or higher in the specific specialty, or its equivalent. H-1B specialty occupations may include fields such as science, engineering and information technology.

Some GME residency programs sponsor H-1B visas for the candidates who have completed all USMLE Steps including Step 3. The major advantage of this visa over J-1 visa is that you are not subjected to 'two-year home return' requirement after the completion of residency training. And hence you do not have to do the J-1 waiver post-residency. However, if you want to do fellowship after residency, very few programs offer H-1B as compared to many programs who offer J-1. Table 11.1 shows the major differences between the two visas.

Table 11.1 Shows major differences between a J-1 visa and a H-1B visa [5]

Features	J-1 visa	H-1B visa
Sponsoring source	ECFMG, Department of State and Homeland Security	Residency program
Requirements	USMLE Step 1, Step 2 CK and CS and ECFMG Certificate	USMLE Step 1, Step 2 CK and CS, Step 3 and ECFMG Certificate
Type of visa	Exchange visitor's visa	Employment visa
Time limit	7 years	6 years (may be extended in certain circumstances)
Fees	$340–$805	$1500–$6000
Processing time	1–2.5 months approx.	Conventional time, 3–5 months Premium processing, 15 days
Mandatory return to home country after residency?	Yes for 2 years, which can be waived by serving for 3 years in a medically underserved area in the United States	No
Spouse and family visa sponsorship	J2 for dependents (spouse and children under 21 years)	H4 for dependents (spouse and children under 21 years)
Can the employer sponsor for US permanent residency?	No	Yes. After residency training, the applicants would need to get a job on H-1B visa and then transit to green card

TABLE 11.1 (continued)

Features	J-1 visa	H-1B visa
Advantages	Easier process Faster and cheaper option Majority of the programs accept this visa	No mandatory home country return after residency More job options to apply for after residency
Disadvantages	Mandatory 2-year home country return or J-1 waiver. Visa stamp needs to be renewed every year at a US consulate outside of the United States	Higher fees for application Very few fellowship programs offer H-1B visa, which narrows the options for fellowship

References

1. https://www.uscis.gov.
2. http://www.usmleweb.com/visa_img.html.
3. https://www.ecfmg.org/evsp/about.html.
4. http://www.rxpgonline.com/article302.html.
5. https://ecuadoctors.com/j1-vs-h1b-visa-residency/.

Part II
Interview

Chapter 12
How to Get a Strong Letter of Recommendation?

Nidhi Shankar Kikkeri and Shivaraj Nagalli

Beauty attracts the eyes but personality captures your heart ~Anonymous

Introduction

In simple words, a letter of recommendation (LoR) is a letter endorsing you for the residency position you are applying. It is a reflection of you in the eyes of other people. A strong letter of recommendation tells about your academic performance as well as reveals your distinguishing personal qualities. Hence, it is one of the important parts of a residency application. This chapter highlights the various steps you need to take as a residency candidate to get a strong letter of recommendation.

N. S. Kikkeri (✉)
Drexel University College of Medicine/Hahnemann University Hospital, Philadelphia, PA, USA

S. Nagalli
Department of Internal Medicine, Yuma Regional Medical Center, Yuma, AZ, USA

© Springer Nature Switzerland AG 2020
R. Govindarajan et al. (eds.), *International Medical Graduate and the United States Medical Residency Application*,
https://doi.org/10.1007/978-3-030-31045-5_12

69

Typical LoR Requirements for Residency Application

Most residency programs request for at least three letters of recommendation with a maximum of four. Also, some programs do ask for the letters of recommendation from specific departments. So, make sure that you go through the application requirements of all the programs you are applying to. Further, if you are applying to multiple specialties, it is advisable to upload specialty specific letters of recommendations to the programs.

The Process of Obtaining a Strong LoR

You need advance planning to get a strong letter of recommendation. One of the first steps to obtain a good LoR is to arrange for clinical rotations in the specialty of your interest. Also, if you have the option to choose your mentors, choose wisely. An ideal recommendation letter is from an individual, who is well-known, recognized and highly respected in the field. Note that the letters of recommendation from university programs have a greater value than the letters from private clinics.

The process of obtaining a strong letter begins with YOU. An applicant who shows consistent enthusiasm and professionalism is more likely to get a strong letter of recommendation. Exhibiting a strong work ethic earns you more points. With this in mind, here are several steps you should take during your clinical rotations to secure an outstanding letter of recommendation. Fig. 12.1 shows positive qualities that can fetch strong LORs.

1. *Be punctual.*

Always be on time, whether you are on in-patient or outpatient rotations. It is one of the first things, your attending will notice.

2. *Show enthusiasm.*

Show genuine enthusiasm in everything you do. Be it a simple task of obtaining the history from a patient or a relatively difficult task of writing a review article, always show that you enjoy what you do.

3. *Be nice.*

Simple gestures like 'Hi' or 'Hello', How are you doing?' and a smile to everybody around you shows that you acknowledge their presence and you care for them.

4. *Be eager to help.*

You come across several situations with the patients or the staff you are working with, where you can be of help. A simple gesture of asking "Do you need any help?" or "How can I help you?" can immediately change a person's perspective of you. The faculty or your mentor is more likely to include this quality of yours and write you a personalized letter.

5. *Get to know your attending, the staff and your co-workers.*

Know your attending on a personal level. Share your educational background and your future aspirations with your

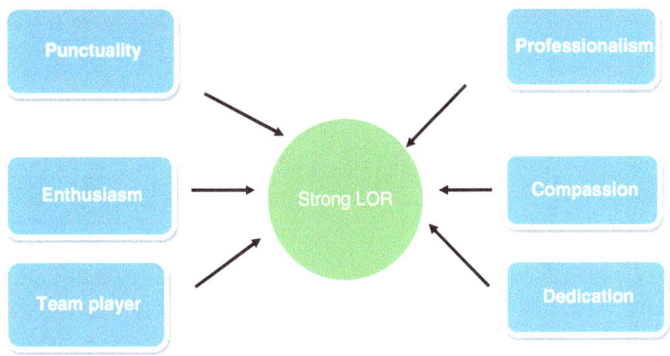

FIGURE 12.1 Shows schematic diagram describing qualities a candidate need to demonstrate to get a strong letter of recommendation

attending. Give them a chance to know who you are as a person. They are more likely to write you a great LoR when they know that you would be a good doctor.

6. *Show attention to detail.*

During your rotations, be very attentive in all the tasks assigned to you. If asked to obtain a history and perform the physical examination, always give your best with close attention to details. This reflects your clinical skills, communication and interpersonal skills.

7. *Ask questions. Do not hesitate.*

After the clinical encounter with the patients, feel free to ask questions to the attending. It shows your genuine interest in the field, your presence of mind and demonstrates that you are eager to learn.

8. *Talk to the residents or fellows.*

Get to know the residents or the fellows in the program, if you are doing rotations in an academic hospital. They can be of extreme help in understanding the residency program dynamics. Express your interest, offer help in doing simple things if allowed to. You can help them in collecting resources for their PowerPoint presentations or research projects. Remember, the residents may provide their valuable input about you to their attending, which may be reflected in the LOR.

Whom to Ask for the Letter?

Letter of recommendation should be requested from the faculty with whom you have worked or done clinical rotations. Request the letter from the physician who knows you well at a personal level, who recognizes your qualities and appreciates you for your work and who believes you would be a good physician. The longer you have worked with a particular attending, the more weightage will be given to the letter from them. Letters obtained from the doctors practicing in the United States have a greater weightage in comparison to the letters obtained from the doctors of your home countries. But, in a scenario, where you fail to obtain any rotations in the United States, you can always use your home country letters of recommendation.

If you have research experience, you can also ask your research mentors to write the letters. These letters can particularly highlight your abilities in conducting research work.

It is not advisable to get letters of recommendation from the residents or your relatives. If you have worked with the residents or spent a considerable amount of time with them during your rotations, you can let your attending know about it. Your attending can get feedback from them and write a strong letter of recommendation for you.

When Is the Ideal Time to Ask for a Letter?

Towards the end of your clinical rotation or soon after the rotation would be an ideal time to request for a LoR. It is this time, the letter author will be able to remember you well and write a better, personalized and a more thorough letter describing your clinical skills, interpersonal skills and your personality.

It is not unusual to request the letter of recommendation several months after clinical rotation as the ERAS token open mid-summer. Hence, while requesting for the letter, it would be appropriate to write a personalized email to your attending describing your past work experience with them, your achievements and your future aspirations. Providing them with a copy of your CV and USMLE transcripts would also be helpful in composing the letter.

Keep in mind that, the letter authors come across several medical students and graduates and will have several requests for writing LoRs. Hence giving them sufficient time after a request is made is necessary. Even after the letter is written and uploaded, ERAS requires 5–7 business days for processing to establish its authenticity before it is released to the residency candidate. Hence, the sooner the better! This way letters can be uploaded in a timely manner.

A letter can be assigned to the residency programs as the fourth LoR at a later date if it is not ready at the beginning of the application season. You can also update the programs through emails if you happen to obtain a stronger letter of recommendation after you have submitted the application through ERAS.

Elements of the Letter of Recommendation

An ideal letter will be written based on the following elements.

1. *Duration of the rotation*:

This would tell the reader where and how long the candidate has worked with the author. Your attending can highlight any specific incidents during your rotation, where you performed really well and stand out from others.

2. *Clinical skills*:

The attending can comment on the candidate's clinical abilities, history taking and skills of performing physical examination. The author can also discuss your bedside manners and your interactions with the patients. Your ability to comprehend information, interpretation of lab values and reaching a differential diagnosis can also be commented on. If you took part in research with your mentor, they can mention it too. This section can show your knowledge of medical literature.

3. *Personal characteristics*:

Here, your mentor can mention about your distinguishing personal qualities like your communication and interpersonal skills, your relation with your co-workers, patients and with the ancillary staff. Your mentor can also talk about your genuine interest in the field, enthusiasm, consistency, motivation, professionalism, and work ethic. Further, it would be advisable to highlight the strong qualities with instances from your rotation to demonstrate the said qualities, rather than blandly listing the qualities. These instances make the letter a personalized one.

4. *Concluding points*:

Here, the letter authors provide their final input and their overall impression of you. They can also discuss the competitiveness of your residency application.

5. *Designation of the author*:

Your letter writers should end the letter with their signature, full name, and designation. They also need to include their contact info such as phone number and an email address.

Should You Waive the Rights to View Your Letter?

Preferably YES! As far as possible, always waive your rights to view your letters of recommendation. A waived letter is perceived as a more honest and reliable description about you than an un-waived letter. However, if you are unsure about your performance during the clinical rotation, it would be in your best interest to view the letter before assigning to the programs. It is always better to assign an un-waived good letter than a mediocre waived letter.

Express Gratitude to Your Letter Writers:

Thank and express gratitude to the letter authors for taking some time off of their busy life to put in words in your favor. Keep them updated during the interview season. You can also send 'Thank You' cards to appreciate their effort in writing LoRs.

Conclusion

A letter of recommendation is a critical component of your residency application. Obtaining a strong letter of recommendation requires advance planning, sincere effort, hard work and persistence from your part. In the end, always give your best during your clinical rotations and aim for a strong personalized letter of recommendation which can help you in securing the position of your choice.

Chapter 13
How to Write
a Competitive Personal
Statement?

Sorabh Datta

> *We do not need magic to transform our world. We carry all*
> *of the power we need inside ourselves already ~J. K. Rowling*

Purpose of Personal Statement

- What is Personal Statement (PS)?
- What is the importance of PS?
- Why it is regarded as the most dreaded aspects of the residency application?
- Why it causes anxiety among the International Medical Graduates (IMGs)?

These are most of the questions we encounter when we start our residency application process. I was in the same position when I began my residency application. All these questions bombarded my mind and trust me it can be really frustrating when you have to put your entire medical career vision into words. But during these tough situations, good ideas knock at your door. So don't worry guys! By the end of

S. Datta (✉)
Pravara Institute of Medical Sciences, Ahmednagar, India

© Springer Nature Switzerland AG 2020
R. Govindarajan et al. (eds.), *International Medical Graduate and the United States Medical Residency Application*,
https://doi.org/10.1007/978-3-030-31045-5_13

77

this chapter, you will feel confident for your PS writing, and you will be able to express your real self in your own PS.

Well PS sometimes also called as a statement of purpose is defined as admissions or application essay written by the residency applicant for getting an interview invite. PS is one aspect of the residency application where you will have complete freedom in expressing yourself and full control over it. So this is the best opportunity for all the residency applicants to impress the selection committee. PS is often considered as pre-interview, as through PS you should be able to answer all the questions of the selection committee before meeting them. Figure 13.1 is an attempt to explain the importance of PS in each specialty [1].

PS can be used by the residency programs in two ways:

1. *Rule in*: To select the ideal candidates which will be a good fit for their programs
2. *Rule out*: To eliminate those individuals who show mistakes like visionless, relatively illiterate, not a good fit in their program

Common Mistakes in PS Writing

- *Avoiding red flags*: Like low USMLE scores, any attempt, long year of graduation, etc. You should address them in your PS and be honest about accepting it.

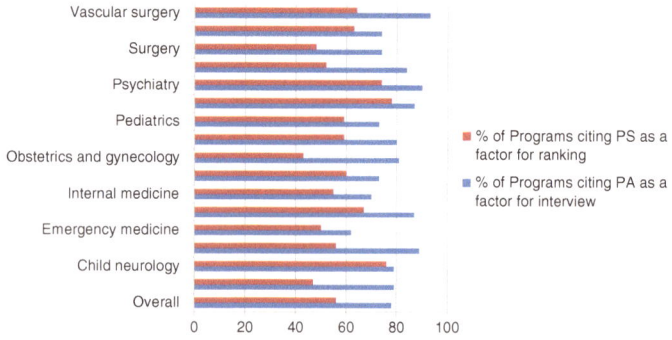

FIGURE 13.1 Shows importance of Personal Statement in specialties for selecting candidates for an interview [1]

- *Repeating too much of your CV*: Remember PS is different from your CV.
- *Sounding like Thesaurus*: Words are too big to understand and use of words which doesn't reflect your personality. You will look artificial to the audience.
- *Too much bragging about yourself*: Being humble in your life is as important as being a responsible resident. So be grounded in your PS.
- *Length issues*: Either too lengthy or too short.
- *Being generic*: If you sound like everyone else, how will you look different from the crowd. So be specific and unique in your PS.
- *Too dramatic*: You are not competing for academy awards here. Be natural and honest in your PS.
- *Grammatical mistakes*: Like spelling mistakes. Remember the first impression is the last impression. Grammar is the most avoidable mistake for anyone.

Rules for Writing Personal Statement

Figure 13.2 explains the structure of a Personal Statement to guide.

- *Never underestimate the importance of the PS*: Individual residency programs assign varying degrees of concern to the PS. Therefore every program has its own significance for the PS. Figure 13.1 shows the importance of the PS as a citing factor for the interview selection and for the ranking.
- *Read the program website before starting with your PS*: Some programs specify to the applicants that what they are looking for in their PS. Before you start, it is right for you to carefully review any personal statement directions mentioned by the residency program. (Yes you can upload different PS for different programs!!)
- *Know your audience*: Read about the Program Director's message on their website, read about the faculty, staff and the residents. Program Director's vision about the program

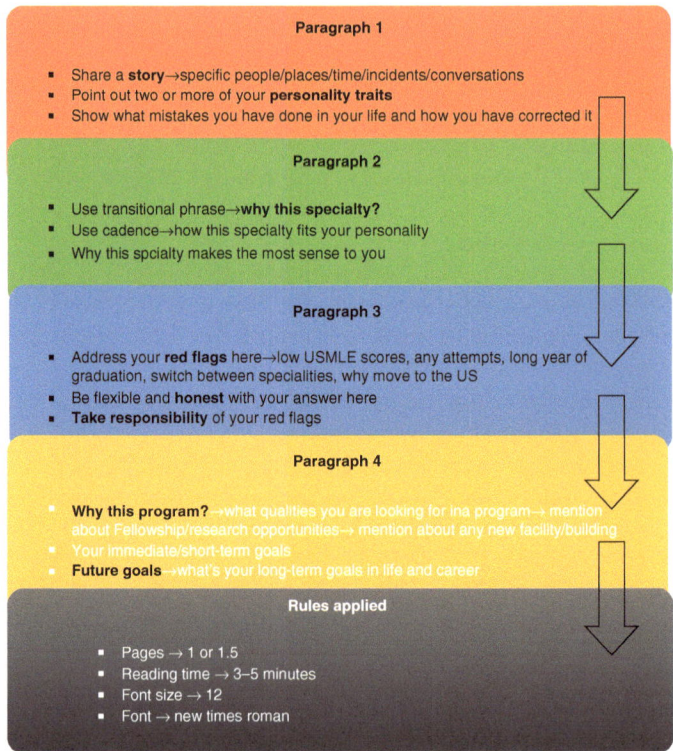

Paragraph 1

- Share a **story**→specific people/places/time/incidents/conversations
- Point out two or more of your **personality traits**
- Show what mistakes you have done in your life and how you have corrected it

Paragraph 2

- Use transitional phrase→**why this specialty?**
- Use cadence→how this specialty fits your personality
- Why this specialty makes the most sense to you

Paragraph 3

- Address your **red flags** here→low USMLE scores, any attempts, long year of graduation, switch between specialities, why move to the US
- Be flexible and **honest** with your answer here
- **Take responsibility** of your red flags

Paragraph 4

- **Why this program?** →what qualities you are looking for in a program→ mention about Fellowship/research opportunities→ mention about any new facility/building
- Your immediate/short-term goals
- **Future goals** →what's your long-term goals in life and career

Rules applied

- Pages → 1 or 1.5
- Reading time → 3–5 minutes
- Font size → 12
- Font → new times roman

FIGURE 13.2 Explains the structure of Personal Statement

sometimes also mentioned on their website. All these things will give you information about your readers. Your ultimate goal is to make a connection with your audience through your PS.

- *Focus more on why this specialty rather than why becoming a physician*: For the residency programs they are more interested in why you have chosen a career in that specialty rather than the reasons that led you to become a physician.
- *Never lie, Never exaggerate*: Don't be a bragger about anything in your life. They are looking for an honest resident who is humble in his/her achievements. One lie can be an

application killer and ultimately killing your dream of being a resident. So be honest and truthful.

- *Don't plagiarize*: A copy cat is a copycat. The residency program has software which can detect the plagiarism if present. This will end your dream as well. Don't use sample PS material given on the internet. You can use them as a guide but don't use their words.
- *Start early, finish early*: You have to be ready with your application by September. So make a deadline for your PS. Remember if you put everything for the end, you will get more anxious and less productive. So don't wait for the last minute.
- *Start your PS with brainstorming*: Take a piece of paper or take your computer and start by making a blueprint of your PS. If you have a plan, you will have a result.
- *Don't be shy from sharing your extraordinary attributes*: If you have a unique skill or achievement, make sure that your audience knows about it. Tell the readers how that skill can be helpful in your future career as a resident in their program.
- *The first draft is the hardest*: Try to make multiple drafts for your PS. The more revisions you will have the more unique your PS will look.
- *The right size does matter for your PS*: Ideally, your reader should be able to read the entire PS in 3–5 minutes. Anything too short or too lengthy will be a negative thing for your PS.
- *Avoid grammatical mistakes*: PS reflects your speaking skills so any single error in the grammar will show your lousy communication skills.
- *Try to not just list your qualities or talents*: Try to correlate what your quality or talent can bring to the program and hospital. For e.g.: mentioning you are good at chess just lists your quality but if you say, strategic and logical thinking acquired as a chess player help me to brainstorm for clinical diagnosis and think two steps ahead, would fetch you more brownie points.

Reference

1. 2018 NRMP Program Director Survey. 2018. www.nrmp.org. Accessed 7 Feb 2019.

Chapter 14
What is MSPE?

Harleen Kaur

> *An Ounce of performance is worth pounds of promises ~Mae West*

Introduction

Medical School Performance Evaluation or initially known as "Dean's Letter" is one of the crucial components of the residency application. The MSPE was introduced by the Association of American Medical Colleges (AAMC) to provide a comprehensive assessment of the applicant's performance in the medical school to the residency program directors. It is mandatory for all residency applicants to submit the MSPE for residency application. According to the AAMC guidelines the MSPE is submitted by the medical schools before the deadline and released to all residency training programs (MD program) on October 1.

H. Kaur (✉)
Adesh Institute of Medical Sciences and Research, Bathinda, India

Department of Neurology, University of Missouri, Columbia, MO, USA
e-mail: kaurha@health.missouri.edu

© Springer Nature Switzerland AG 2020   83
R. Govindarajan et al. (eds.), *International Medical Graduate and the United States Medical Residency Application*,
https://doi.org/10.1007/978-3-030-31045-5_14

Content of the Letter

The MSPE usually include professional and personal background of the applicant reflecting his/her undergraduate performance. There is a standardized MSPE generated by the schools based on the AAMC guidelines as shown in Fig. 14.1. The clinical performance of the applicant included in the MSPE is based on the Objective Structural Clinical Examination (OSCE) taken during the medical school. The MSPE also includes charts and histograms to depict the ranking of the students in comparison to other classmates. This is helpful for competitive programs and helps them to stand out. The MSPEs also include information about honors, awards, class ranks and other curricular and volunteer activities. Most medical schools do not share information about the applicants failing grades, borderline performance, leaves or absence, as it would reflect on their own program as well. Most of the time the applicant gets a chance to review the MSPE thoroughly before submitting it the Electronic Residency Application System (ERAS). A sample format of the MSPE is shown in Fig. 14.2.

AAMC recommendation for writing MSPE

1.The information provided in the MSPE should be clear, concise and standardized.

2.Explain the MSPE in six sections including Identifying Information, Noteworthy Characteristics, Academic History, Academic Progress, summary and Medical School Information.

3.The six American Council of Graduate Medical Education (ACGME) core competencies should be highlighted, if mentioned.

4.Explain applicants' academic performance in medical school including details of professionalism.

5. Include 'Noteworthy Characteristics' instead of 'Unique Characteristics'.

6. Include Comparative data in the form of charts or histograms and how this information is derived.

7. Define overall rating and adjectives if used.

8. The MSPE should not exceed seven pages and should be typed in 12-point single spaced font.

FIGURE 14.1 AAMC Guidelines for writing MSPE

School of Medicine Date

IDENTIFYING INFORMATION

<Student's legal name and year in school name and location of medical school>

NOTEWORTHY CHARACTERISTICS

<Provide a maximum of three characteristics highlighting the most salient noteworthy characteristics of the student. This section should be presented as a bulleted list. Each characteristic should be described in 2 sentences or less. Information about any significant challenges or hardships encountered by the student during medical school may be included.>

- <text>
- <text>
- <text>

ACADEMIC HISTORY

Date of Initial Matriculation in Medical School	
Date of Expected Graduation from Medical School	
Please explain any extensions, leave(s), gap(s), or break(s) in the student's educational program below:	
Information about the student's prior, current, or expected enrollment in, and the month and year of the student's expected graduation from dual, joint or combined degree programs.	
Was the student required to repeat or otherwise remediate any course work during their medical education? If yes, please explain.	
Was the student the recipient of any adverse action(s) by the medical school or its parent institution?	

ACADEMIC PROGRESS

Professional Performance

<Describe how the medical school defines professionalism and what it assesses in students. Whenever possible, areas of strength and weakness should be addressed.>

Preclinical Coursework

<If preclinical courses are graded as Pass/Fail, the MSPE should convey that the student has met all requirements. Whenever possible, areas of strength and weakness should be addressed.>

Clerkships (in chronological order)

<The components of each clerkship grade and the weight of each component (for example, % clinical assessment, % shelf exam, % case write-up, % OSCE, etc.) should be included to better inform program directors on performance. Whenever possible, areas of strength and weakness should be addressed. Clerkship evaluations are a crucial piece of information for program directors and are considered by many to be the most important section of the MSPE in determining applicants for interview selection and rank order list.>

NOTE: The graphs included in this template are meant **only** as examples. Schools should use their own grading systems or schemes in their graphs depicting comparative student performance.

FIGURE 14.2 Sample MSPE format according to AAMC guidelines. (Courtesy: AAMC website [1])

Specialty Month-Month Year Grade: Overall Grade based on

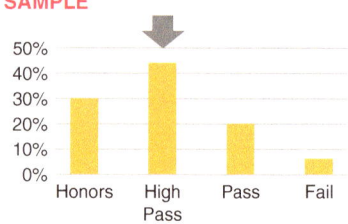

Specialty Month-Month Year Grade: Overall Grade based on\<text\>

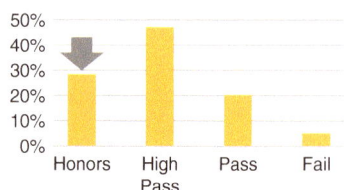

Specialty Month-Month Year Grade: Overall Grade based on\<text\>

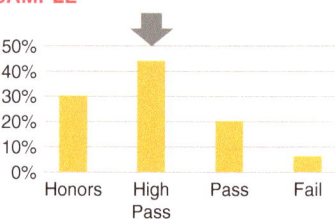

Specialty Month-Month Year Grade: Overall Grade based on\<text\>

SUMMARY

\<The Task Force recommends providing a summative assessment, based upon the school's evaluation system, of the student's comparative performance in medical school, relative to their peers. Schools should include information about any school-specific categories used in differentiating among levels of student performance. This may, though does not have to, include graphic

Representation of the student's performance relative to their class overall\>

Sincerely,

FIGURE 14.2 (continued)

MSPE for Foreign Medical Graduates (FMG)

Most foreign medical schools are aware of the MSPE, and have a set format that abides by the AAMC guidelines. Since it is the applicant's responsibility to ask for the MSPE, it is best to reach the Dean's office ahead of time, and get the documents ready by the deadline date. The format of the MSPE may vary from that of the US medical schools but it is crucial to include all important information in your MSPE as summarized in Fig. 14.2.

Conclusion

MSPE is an important requirement for the residency application and provides useful information regarding the applicant's academic performance. Applicants, especially foreign medical graduates are required to collect all the valid information way before time, in order to complete the MSPE and submit it to ERAS on time. MSPE along with other source of assessment like the transcripts, résumé are important sources to evaluate the applicants, hence should be reviewed thoroughly and submitted on time.

Reference

1. www.aamc.org.

Chapter 15
How Can I Make My CV Strong?

Nidhi Shankar Kikkeri and Shivaraj Nagalli

Every accomplishment starts with a decision to try
~Anonymous

Introduction

Curriculum Vitae (CV) is a vital document consisting of a comprehensive description of one's background, academic credentials, achievements, work and volunteer experiences. The goal of a CV is to provide the reader with a summary of your accomplishments while seeking for a job in any field. The CV is typically the first document used by the residency programs to review your residency application. A strong CV is vital in creating a good first impression and can get you an interview. This chapter highlights the ways to write an impressive CV for the residency application.

N. S. Kikkeri (✉)
Drexel University College of Medicine/Hahnemann University Hospital, Philadelphia, PA, USA

S. Nagalli
Department of Internal Medicine, Yuma Regional Medical Center, Yuma, AZ, USA

© Springer Nature Switzerland AG 2020   89
R. Govindarajan et al. (eds.), *International Medical Graduate and the United States Medical Residency Application*,
https://doi.org/10.1007/978-3-030-31045-5_15

Why Do I Need a CV?

You need a CV to:

- Apply for the electives, observerships and externships.
- Provide as a reference to the mentors who write your letters of recommendation.
- Apply to the residency programs participating in the match.
- Apply to the residency programs which do not take part in the match.

How Long Should My CV Be?

It is not the length of your CV, but the content that matters. Depending on the number of work and research experiences, the length of the CV can vary. While preparing a CV, the goal should be to convey the programs why you would be a suitable candidate for the program and how you are better than the others. It is advisable to be concise and precise.

What's the Best CV Format?

While writing the CV, organizing the information in different sections in the reverse chronological order is recommended. That is to start with what you are doing currently and work backward.

Elements of a CV

1. *Personal information*:

Give your full name exactly as it appears in your medical school records. Provide your current home address and telephone number, where you can be reached in case the programs want to contact you. A valid email address is mandatory as most of the programs communicate and correspond through emails.

2. *Education*:

Include the name of your medical school and the duration of training, specifying the year of graduation. If you have completed postgraduate training, you can include that as well.

3. *Professional society memberships*:

If you are a member of any professional organizations, you can list your memberships here.

4. *Awards and accomplishments*:

Here, you can list any academic or community awards received till date. It can be during your medical school or after. You can include prizes won in the competitions during the medical schooling. You should be able to judge, whether your achievements are valuable to your application.

5. *Volunteer experience*:

You can write about your volunteer experiences during your medical school or after you graduated. This section highlights your commitment to the community you lived in. This can also include your leadership roles if you have held any. Also, remember a lot of volunteer experience can help an application to family medicine programs or internal medicine programs in the rural communities, but might not be that valuable for the surgical residency programs.

6. *Work experience*:

As mentioned earlier, this consists of the work experience which is to be written in the reverse chronological order. Here, you should include all your rotations, electives, observerships and externships. List your position, the duration and your mentor for each work experience. You can elaborate on your role and the activities you took part during the rotations. You can describe the experience either in paragraphs or bulletin points. Remember, space is limited for each experience. So, try to be concise and provide valuable information.

7. *Research experience*:

Write about your position, duration of research, where you performed it and under whose guidance. You can elaborate on your role in the research, the goal and the outcome. Be aware of what you are writing, as you can be asked questions about any part of the research you have mentioned in an interview.

8. *Publications and presentations*:

You can list the papers that you have worked on, published or presented by the title and the date of publication or presentation. If you have presented posters at national level or state level conferences, you must include it here. While mentioning publications, remember there are different options like submitted, provisionally accepted and published. Be honest and cite your publications appropriately. The programs can verify the status of your articles. Hence, do not include any false information.

9. *Hobbies and interests*:

List your hobbies and interests in this section. Again, you can opt to write in the form of a paragraph or in bulletin points. Be genuine and mention what you really like to do. Avoid portraying yourself as something you are not.

10. *Language fluency*:

You can list the languages you speak and describe your proficiency in each one of them.

Tips to Remember (as Shown in Fig. 15.1)

- Your CV should be concise, easy to read and in an organized format.
- The person who reads your CV should get a brief idea about who you are from your CV. This person might not

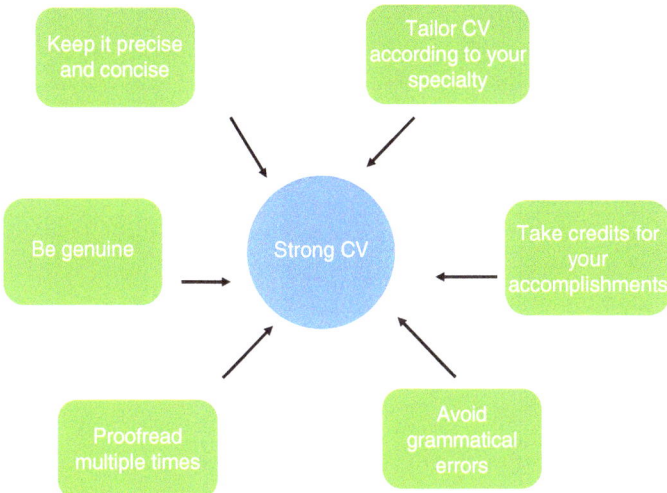

FIGURE 15.1 Shows schematic diagram describing the tips to make a strong CV

have a lot of time to spend on reading each application completely. So, be precise.

- Be accurate while presenting your work experiences. Reverse chronological order is recommended while presenting this information.
- Avoid grammatical errors and spelling mistakes. Such mistakes may reflect poor language skills and can be detrimental to your residency application.
- Proofread your final CV multiple times before submitting. It is also advisable to get your final CV proofread by your mentors or other professionals aware of the residency application.
- Be genuine while providing the information. Also, note that you can be questioned about any information in your CV. So, be prepared to talk on everything that is included in your CV if selected for an interview.
- Do not falsify any part of your CV including work experiences or publications.

- If you are applying to one specialty, try to tailor your CV toward that specialty. Stress on the work experiences in that particular specialty.
- If you are applying to multiple specialties, be careful when you are listing work experiences and publications. You are more likely to get interviews from the specialty where you have had more work experience.
- Take credit for everything you have accomplished. This is your chance to show the programs what you are capable of and how you can contribute.

Conclusion

Curriculum Vitae is an essential component of the residency application. A poorly written CV can eliminate your application from the interview selection process. So, spend enough time when you prepare your CV. Be precise and specific while presenting the information. Remember, your goal should be to come up with an impressive CV, which can convince the reader that you are the person they are looking for!

There are many sample CVs which you can come across online; we have a sample CV as shown in Figs. 15.2, 15.3 and 15.4. Again note, do not copy any CV from across the Internet. It is considered plagiarism. They are just there for you to know the style of writing and to give you a clue as to how it should be presented.

SAMPLE CV

FIRST NAME MIDDLE LAST NAME

PERSONAL INFORMATION

ADDRESS
PHONE NUMBER
E-MAIL

AAMC ID:

ACADEMICS

COURSE	BOARDS/UNIVERSITY	SCORE, YEAR OF PASSING
Secondary School Certificate	Central Board of Secondary Education	97%; 2002
Higher School Certificate	Central Board of Secondary Education	94%; 2004

MEDICAL EDUCATION

MBBS (Bachelor of Medicine and Bachelor of Surgery)	2004-2010
YMSD Medical College and Research institute	
Under Rajiv Gandhi University of Health Sciences	

Education Commission for Foreign Medical Graduates (ECFMG) Certification	Feb 2011

CURRENT ACTIVITY

Research Assistant, Department of Nephrology Univeristy of Pittsburgh, Pittsburgh, April 2012-Present PA
Clinical observer, Nephrology under Dr Mefooz Anand, University of Pittsburgh, PA April 2012-Present

FIGURE 15.2 Showing a sample CV, page 1

USMLE SCORES

Step 1:	260 (Pass)	August 2010
Step 2:	265 (Pass)	January 2011
Step 2CS:	PASS (1st Attempt)	Feb 2011
Step 3:	232	April 2012

US CLINICAL EXPERIENCE

Clinical Observer Department of Cardiology, Univeristy of Chicago, Illinois	March 2011-May 2011
Clinical Observer Department of Rheumatology, Washington University, St Louis, MO	August 2011-May 2011
Clinical Observer Department of Pulmonary Medicine, University of Pittsburgh, Pittsburgh, PA	Dec 2011-March 2012

RESEARCH EXPERIENCES

Case Report: [TITLE OF CASE REPORT]: Authors with [Last name, First name], [Name of journal] (published) [source/link]
May 2011

Review Article: [TITLE OF REVIEW ARTICLE]: Authors with [Last name, First name], [Name of journal] (accepted for publication)
Aug 2011

Research Paper: [TITLE OF RESEARCH PAPER]: Authors with [Last name, First name], [Name of journal] (submitted)
Sept 2011

Retrospective review: [TITLE OF RETROSPECTIVE REVIEW]: Authors with [Last name, First name], (Under Preparation)
April 2012

HONORS AND ACHIEVEMENT

Secured Gold Medal in Physiology and Pathology in MBBS under RGUHS	2006
Scholarship for being in top 1% for National level Pathology Quiz	2006
Secured Distinction (equivalent to honors) in all 4 years of MBBS	2010

FIGURE 15.3 Showing a sample CV, page 2

CLINICAL EXPERIENCE

Worked under Dr Gliazeh Gomez (MBBS, MD, MRCP) in Department of Medicine   Apr 2010-May2011
Apollo Hospital, INDIA

VOLUNTEER ACTIVITY

Participated in Stroke Awareness Program under Department of Neurology where performed free risk
assessment screening and generate awareness about stroke.   March 2012

Participated in Multiple vaccination camps where we went house to house to deliver vaccination and health
education under Dr Bal, Head of Department, Dept of Community Medicine   2004-2010

Assisted and participated in paediatric healthcare in rural population under Dr Hanz, Chief Medical
officer, Rural Jaipur, India.   Apr 2009-Aug 2009

EXTRACURRICULAR ACTIVITIES

Mention your hobbies (Please do not mention watching TV as hobby)
any sports/cultural events participation and prize
Any designing/leadership skills

FIGURE 15.4 Showing a Sample CV-Page 3

Chapter 16
I Got an Interview, How Do I Prepare for It?

Nidhi Shankar Kikkeri and Shivaraj Nagalli

Success is where preparation and opportunity meet ~ Anonymous

Introduction

Congratulations! You have been selected for an interview.

Receiving a residency interview invite itself is an achievement and is highly exciting for any residency candidate. This is a sign that the residency program is impressed by your application. Now, it is time to impress the interview committee in person. So, put your best effort to ace the interview. This chapter highlights the steps to prepare well for an interview.

N. S. Kikkeri (✉)
Drexel University College of Medicine/Hahnemann University Hospital, Philadelphia, PA, USA

S. Nagalli
Department of Internal Medicine, Yuma Regional Medical Center, Yuma, AZ, USA

© Springer Nature Switzerland AG 2020
R. Govindarajan et al. (eds.), *International Medical Graduate and the United States Medical Residency Application*,
https://doi.org/10.1007/978-3-030-31045-5_16

Practice Makes You Perfect

As with any skill or expertise, the more we practice, the better we get at it. Yes, to ace the interview, we do need proper preparation and practice. Do not wait till the last minute to start preparing for your interview. Plan ahead and start early. Practice will instill confidence and reduce the anxiety on your big day. It will make you calmer and appear more organized and presentable in the real interview.

One of the best ways to practice is through mock interviews. A mock interview is a simulation of an interview intended for training purpose. It helps in identifying your weak areas through honest and valuable feedback from the interviewers. Hence, these mock interviews should be as realistic as possible to give you a real interview experience. They can also be helpful in learning various ways to tackle tough and unfamiliar questions. The mentors who have experience in conducting the interviews would be better in judging your performance. You can also approach resident physicians to conduct mock interviews. In case you do not have mentors or residents, you can always practice with other candidates in the same boat. Be open to their suggestions and advise.

One of the useful techniques for self-critique is to video record your mock interview. The video can allow you to judge your performance better. It lets you visualize your body language and communication skills, which are very important for an interview.

When you are practicing the answers for interview questions, one important thing to remember is not to memorize the answers. The interviewers do not like to listen to rehearsed answers. The programs prefer candidates who are spontaneous and natural. So keep this in mind when you practice. You can instead prepare a list of points for each of the common interview questions and can talk naturally on those points.

Know the Program

Once you get an interview, you need to start researching the program thoroughly. You should try to know everything about the program and the city where you might be spending the next 3–4 years of your life.

When you are gathering information about the programs, look for the strengths and weaknesses of every program where you will be interviewing. If you are a research-oriented candidate, you may want to find out if the particular program offers enough research opportunities to reach your full potential. Some of the university programs tend to emphasize more on research compared to smaller community programs. Also, look into the location where the program is located and various outdoor activities and things that the city has to offer during your residency. This can help you in answering the common interview question, "Why do you want to be in our program?"

Most programs will have a good online website with details about various clinical sites of teaching, the curriculum, the faculty, the current residents, available fellowship opportunities, and resident fellowship matching rates. If programs have minimal information on their website, you need to look for alternate sources to gather the data. Reaching out to your friends or medical school seniors who might be current residents or recent graduates from the program where you will be interviewing can be beneficial. They can provide valuable information about the program which may not be listed on the online resources.

You can also look up the research work or publications of the faculty who will be interviewing you. This might reveal some of the common areas of research you might share with them and you can talk about it in detail during the interview. This is a nice way to develop a good rapport with your interviewer and express your interest to work with them in the future.

Pre-interview dinners are nice opportunities to learn more about the program from the residents in an informal environment. The residents tend to give you more honest and better input on the teaching, faculty, and the resident schedules.

What Should I Be Prepared for?

You need to be prepared for everything that is there in your residency application. You never know what can be appealing in your application for the interviewer.

Personal Statement

A lot of questions can be derived from what is written in your personal statement. The discussion can begin with a story you might have shared, your future goals, or anything that might be interesting in it. Many candidates tend to neglect the personal statement. Hence, be prepared for the potential questions from your personal statement.

Work Experience

Know in-depth about your entire work experience including clinical rotations, observerships, or externships. Questions can be directed to describe your clinical work with a particular mentor or a physician or can be generalized to explain the things you have done since the time of graduation from medical school. In general, you can talk about how long you worked with a particular mentor, what were your duties during the rotation, and what you learned from these rotations. Questions regarding your volunteer experiences are also equally important and are frequently asked. Further, be ready to talk about the rotations you have been doing since the time of submission of your application.

Research Experience

Importance of knowing thoroughly about your participation or any involvement in research activity mentioned in the residency application cannot be undermined. Questions can be directed toward your role and the goal of your research work and its outcome. You can also be asked to present a case from one of your articles. Always remember the names of the different journals where your articles have been published or submitted.

Hobbies

Programs also would like to know the interviewees outside of their work. Be genuine and honest when you mention your hobbies in the application. You should be able to engage in a conversation about your likes. The interviewers can easily identify candidates who are portraying themselves as something which they are not.

Common Questions

Apart from what is there in your application, some of the common questions which may be asked in the interviews are listed below:

• Tell me about yourself.
• How did you develop an interest in this specialty?
• Where do you see yourself 10 years down the lane?
• Why do you want to be in our program?
• What are you looking for in a program?
• Why should we choose you over other candidates?
• What are your strengths or weaknesses?
• What can you contribute to our program?
• What do you like to do for fun?
• Tell me about something that is not there in your CV.

- Tell me about an interesting case you have encountered during your rotations. It is always advisable to prepare two to three interesting cases. The interviewer is trying not only to see how you present the case but also what you did and what thought process you had when you were encountered with such a case. So preparing beforehand will help you to be fluent without missing any key point relevant to the case.

Interview Attire

The interview attire can speak volumes about your personality. Dress appropriately to make the best first impression. If you have multiple interviews, it is advisable to have two sets of professional attire.

Pre-interview Dinner

Pre-interview dinner is a semi-formal gathering where you get to meet the other applicants and the residents. This is an opportunity for you to get to know more about the program. You can wear the "business casual" attire for the pre-interview dinners. Men can wear a nice button-up shirt and dark slacks or khaki pants. Sneakers and jeans are to be avoided and wearing a tie is not necessary. Women can wear a nice blouse and slacks or appropriate length skirts. Make sure your clothes are not too provocative or short or display too much skin. Be conservative in dressing yet professional. Also, keep the weather in mind. Candidates with interviews in the east coast should be prepared for the snowy winters.

Interview Day

"Business formal" is the perfect attire for the interview day. Make sure your clothes fit you well and you are comfortable.

Tips for Men

A professional suit is the standard with a nice button-up shirt. The suit can be black, gray, or navy blue.

Wear a tie, but avoid flashy colors.

Wear black or dark brown shoes and clean socks. Make sure your shoes are polished and comfortable to walk during the hospital tour.

Limit jewelry to a watch and a wedding band if you are married.

Avoid strong cologne or deodorants.

Be sure to shave before your interviews, and if you have long hair, get a haircut.

You can carry a folder or a portfolio with a pen to take down notes on the interview day.

Tips for Women

A professional suit is the standard. It can be a pantsuit or a skirt suit. It can be black, gray, or navy blue. Make sure that the skirt extends just below the knees. Avoid flashy colors and miniskirts!

The top you wear under the suit should be in a solid color that complements the suit. Make sure the neckline is not too low.

Wear closed-toe comfortable shoes. If you are comfortable in heels, you can wear them, but remember, you have to walk a lot on the interview day.

Wear limited jewelry. You can wear a watch, simple earrings or studs, a simple necklace, and a wedding band if you are married.

Avoid strong perfumes or deodorants.

Light makeup is acceptable. Avoid dark lipsticks and bright eye shadows. Remember you are going for a residency interview, not a date!

Nails should be trimmed. You can use clear nail polish. Avoid fancy colors.

Hairstyle should be conservative in appearance. Make sure your hair doesn't cover your eyes.

You can have a simple black bag with a zipper to carry your essential items. Avoid big tote bags or backpacks.

You can carry a simple portfolio or a folder with a pen to take down notes.

Travel Arrangements

Travel planning is an essential part of interview preparation and does take time and effort. Hence, you must start planning soon after you get your interview date. If you have to travel for the interviews by flight, it is advisable to book the tickets early to get better deals.

Attending interviews can be a costly affair. If you have the option of clustering interviews geographically over a certain period of time, use it. This would not only allow the trips to be economical but also prevents fatigue due to frequent long-distance travels. However, a word of caution is not to over-burden yourself with multiple back-to-back interviews.

Plan your stay according to your preference and convenience. When you are booking hotels, try to look for places close to your interview locations, so that you are not stuck in traffic and end up late to the interview. If your family or friends stay close by, you can plan to stay with them. Airbnb is another cost-effective option.

Chapter 17
How Many Interviews Do I Need to Be Safe? Is It Same for Prelim and Advanced Programs?

Lakshmi P. Digala

Always hope, but never expect things would go your side every time
~Anonymous

The main motive of an interview for the residency is what a program wanted to know an applicant beyond his/her medical school accomplishments, transcripts, USMLE scores, and letters of recommendation. Henceforth, a huge weight is given for an interview as the program director or the interview faculties are determined to know the following aspects of an applicant [1]:

- Applicant's values and motives toward patient care.
- Professional hopes and dreams.
- Determine if the applicant is a perfect fit.

This is a great opportunity for an applicant themselves after having gone through the entire interview process which is typical almost in every program which ends with a tour, gives an opportunity to envision themselves as a resident in

L. P. Digala (✉)
University of Missouri, Columbia, MO, USA

© Springer Nature Switzerland AG 2020   107
R. Govindarajan et al. (eds.), *International Medical Graduate and the United States Medical Residency Application*,
https://doi.org/10.1007/978-3-030-31045-5_17

that program. The above described motives apply the same to preliminary positions as well as advanced programs.

Contiguous Ranking

When it comes to the number of interviews, an applicant must have to be matched safely. Let's discuss briefly contiguous ranking. Contiguous ranking means the applicant's program rank order list having programs of the same desired specialty before they rank other specialties. Figure 17.1 shows the median number of contiguous ranks of different specialties in 2018.

NRMP data suggest that the more applicants rank programs of their desired specialty, the higher are the chances of matching outcome. In Fig. 17.1, we showed the median number of the contiguous ranking of both US IMGs and non-US IMGs median contiguous ranking [2]. US and non-US IMGs

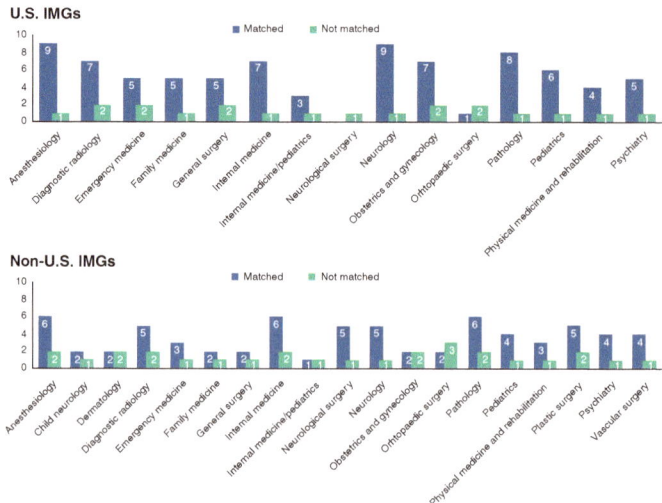

FIGURE 17.1 Shows median number of contiguous ranks of IMG as per 2018 NRMP data by preferred specialty and match outcome [2]

who matched to their preferred specialties have longer contiguous rank lists than those who did not match in almost all specialties. Also, we notice that the rank lists are shorter for US IMGs than non-US IMGs in many specialties.

However, when the applicants rank other programs interspersed with other specialties the chances of match outcome are not as good as with contiguous ranking. Despite all the calculated data, there is no magic number to be safe. The risk of matching is low with a small rank list, and the average rank list number of who matched ranges from 7 to 10.

References

1. https://www.residencyinterviewquestions.com.
2. http://www.nrmp.org/wp-content/uploads/2018/06/Charting-Outcomes-in-the-Match-2018-IMGs.pdf.

Chapter 18
I Have Not Gotten Any Interview, What Should I Do?

Lakshmi P. Digala

We must accept finite disappointment but never lose infinite hope
MLK Jr

The most challenging time of the entire journey to your residency is when a season ends up without any interview. We recommend this is the time for self-reflection of your application before you even start applying next season. By doing this, your goal is to determine if there any red flags and how to overcome them. And, to improve your chances for the next match season.

Many applicants are in the same pool as yours; as per data since 2004, the number of applicants is increasing for an almost similar number of positions making this match even more competitive [1]. In 2018, the number of applicants registering reached an all-time high of 43,909 and active applicants of 37,103, which is 752 more registrants and 1134 more active applicants compared to 2017, as depicted in Fig. 18.1 [2].

There could be several criteria from the program's perspective or reasons from the applicant's end that might result in not securing even an interview spot. Let us discuss in detail those reasons as it gives a chance to work on them. Let us first

L. P. Digala (✉)
University of Missouri, Columbia, MO, USA

© Springer Nature Switzerland AG 2020   111
R. Govindarajan et al. (eds.), *International Medical Graduate and the United States Medical Residency Application*,
https://doi.org/10.1007/978-3-030-31045-5_18

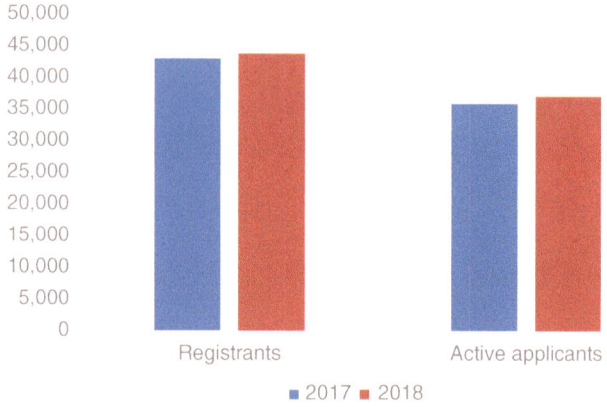

FIGURE 18.1 Rise in number of applicants from 2017 to 2018 Match according to NRMP data

focus on the reasons from applicant's end and below are the topmost reasons for not securing an interview [3]:

- Poor personal statement
- Defective letters of recommendation
- Insufficient US clinical experience
- Poor My ERAS application
- Low scores or attempts
- Incompatible programs
- Incompatible specialty
- Applying delay
- Number of programs applied
- Follow-up with the programs

In the reasons mentioned above, we can classify them as modifiable and non-modifiable, as described in the table below. The factors like the year of graduation, USMLE scores, or any attempts are non-modifiable; hence, pay less focus on them as we cannot change anything. Instead, defective non-modifiable factors that pull down your application could be overcome by working on modifiable factors like letters of recommendation, ERAS application, and personal statement, as shown in Fig. 18.2.

Non-modifiable factors	Modifiable factors
Year of graduation USMLE scores Any attempts in steps	Personal statement Letters of recommendation US clinical experience Research and publishing

FIGURE 18.2 Shows number of modifiable and non-modifiable risk factors

Personal Statement

The first and foremost part of your application is the personal statement. Many applicants give very low priority in drafting the statement of purpose and undermine its importance. We reinforce that in your application packet, this is the first interaction of the program with you. It must be drafted with complete attention as it weighs as an essential part of the application, and it reflects what you are as a person.

Don't rewrite your CV in your statement and always remember to include what attracted to the specialty you are applying to. Also, include why you like the program and create a personalized statement that creates a positive impact on the selection committee. Try to personalize your statement of purpose to every program you are applying, and it is worth spending time on this.

Letter of Recommendation

The second most important part of an application is letters of recommendation, and being an IMG, it becomes even more critical to obtain letters from the US physicians. These letters from them reflect your work in US healthcare setting. That is what a program looks for in your application. The letters obtained from academic hospitals are weighed over letters obtained from privately practicing physicians.

One key rule to keep in mind while you start obtaining them is time. These physicians are already busy in their day-to-day schedule, so give them ample time to work on your letter and follow up on them. It is quite a daunting task getting them uploaded, but make sure you don't rush them as we don't want to create any inconvenience to them. Also, make sure the letters are specific to the specialty you are applying to. The letter is only considered strong if it comes from a physician of the same specialty. The key points to remember about the letters that are weighed highly are:

- Physician of a US teaching hospital
- More recently written
- Specialty specific

US Clinical Experience

Being an IMG set you back over an American medical graduate in the competition as they are well versed in the system. Henceforth, tremendous effort must be put forth to gain US clinical experience may it be the form of away electives or clerkships as medical students. If already graduated, observership or externships can be obtained. Also, any volunteering opportunities or research options must be considered because gaining US clinical experience will boost your resume.

If you have already done such observership/clerkship/externships, take some time to inspect if the length of experience is enough or if you had done the same specialty you are applying to? Your goal out of this experience must not only gaining clinical knowledge but also good letters of recommendation.

Specialty and Program Choice

Picking a specialty should be done smartly, which increases your chance of getting matched, so determine which specialty is right for you. Applying to IMG-friendly specialties increases your chances of getting matched. The top 6 IMG-friendly specialties as per 2018 match data are shown in Fig. 18.3 [4]:

Also, research if the specialty-specific program you are applying is IMG friendly. Let us not waste the resources and effort, hoping to hear from a program which does not consider international graduates. It is time to check if your application meets minimum requirements of the program like

- Visa status
- Attempts in steps
- Minimum score requirements
- ECFMG certification
- Time since graduation

Usually, programs look favorably toward applications that meet their minimum requirements. Even though it is a quite

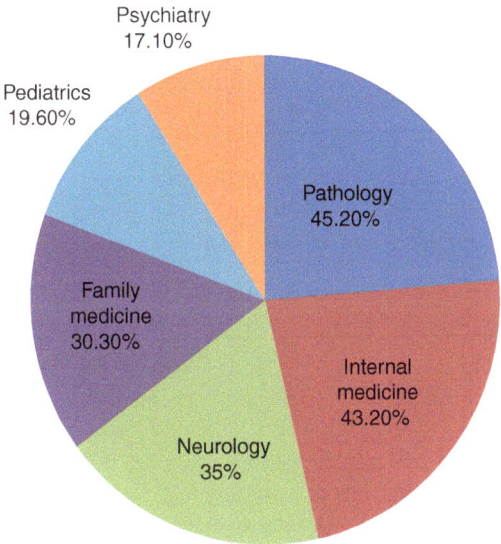

FIGURE 18.3 Top 6 specialties IMG got matched as per NRMP 2018 data. Note: the following data does not consider the total number of residency spots into consideration. It just depicts how many IMGs have matched into the specialty

daunting task to make your application package specific to program, it is the best way to get the attention of the screening persons.

Number of Programs Applied

One big suggestion is to question yourself if you had applied to enough programs to secure you an interview. According to the research, the good number is 100 if the specialty is big enough to improve your probability of getting an interview [3].

Follow-Up

Nevertheless, do not sit back, assuming you will be called for an interview. There is no harm in contacting the program if you do not hear back from them. Many applicants have secured interview spots just by making a phone call or emailing the program reiterating your interest. This only gives a positive outlook of your interest in them from your end. However, remember not to overdo it. Decent communications refer to once in 2 weeks and never forget to mention your AAMC ID in the communication.

Miscellaneous

Research opportunities like data collection, writing case reports, and publishing papers will boost your resume. Look out for opportunities like this in academic institutions may it be university hospitals or community programs. It can be achieved by contacting the programs of your chosen specialty and trying to contact people who are active in research. Finally, never underestimate the importance of personal connections. All sorts of clinical experience mentioned in the chapter above could be easily obtained if you have any personal connections in the program.

After making all the above efforts, make sure you apply on time, and it can be an advantage if you can find a mentor who had already been through this. Their suggestions from their experience are very invaluable. We hope with all these tips you secure an interview for the next match season.

References

1. https://residentsmedical.com.
2. http://www.nrmp.org/main-residency-match-data/.
3. http://blog.matcharesident.com/why-didnt-i-match-14-reasons-you-could-have-failed-to-match/.
4. http://blog.matcharesident.com/top-5-img-friendly-specialties-2018-match/.

Chapter 19
Tips About the Travel Preparation for Interviews

Harleen Kaur

> *Success is a journey, not a destination. The doing is often more important than the outcome ~Anonymous*

Introduction

Travelling during interview season can be cumbersome, tiring, and expensive, but at the same time, it is an opportunity to see and explore different parts of the country. The interview season occurs during the unpredictable weather conditions which can result in frequent delays or cancellation of flights and uncomfortable accommodation. Also, this time of the year is considered as the holiday season from Thanksgiving to Christmas and Hanukah, which anticipates increase in number of frequent flyers and expensive flights booking. The cost of travelling during this time can be burdensome as well. It is estimated that an average medical

———
H. Kaur (✉)
Adesh Institute of Medical Sciences and Research, Bathinda, India

Department of Neurology, University of Missouri,
Columbia, MO, USA
e-mail: kaurha@health.missouri.edu

© Springer Nature Switzerland AG 2020   119
R. Govindarajan et al. (eds.), *International Medical Graduate and the United States Medical Residency Application*,
https://doi.org/10.1007/978-3-030-31045-5_19

student spends roughly 4000$–15,000$ on travel and lodging during interviews. In order to reduce this cost of trip, some people also prefer to organize their interview in clusters. Having interviews in coordinated dates definitely helps to cut down the cost of travelling, but at the same time, it may get hectic and tiring, and there may also be time constraints when gathering all the information about the program. Managing the travel during interview in the right way can help to reduce a lot of stress related to the interview. This chapter aims to overcome the stress related to travelling and understand the minute details that can be helpful in travel preparation.

Packing

Always prefer a carry-on baggage over check-in baggage. Make sure you keep all the travel documents handy. Also, keep copy of your ticket, accommodation, venue location and airline helpline number in hand. It is always preferable to pack your interview dress/suit and pre-interview dress in the carry-on baggage. All the packing items including the pants, shirts, jackets, dress, and blouses should be zipped and buttoned and placed side to side in the suitcase alternating on each other. Every item should be folded along their natural seems one on top of other to cushion one another and keep them neat and without creases. Packing the clothes separately in plastic cleaner's bag can also help to keep them clean and neat. It is also advisable to first place a layer of t-shirts, sleepwear and sweaters in the suitcase and then place the interview suit over it as discussed. The toiletries, socks, shoes, belts and any other accessories can be rolled on the sides of the suitcase. Cover the entire pile with a large towel and then secure it with suitcase belts. Also, plan to carry all electronic devices like iPad, laptop in a separate laptop bag along with their chargers. Lastly, make a travel checklist and go over to make sure you have packed everything.

Mode of Communication/Travelling

Most applicants plan to travel by air for the interviews. However, rental cars, buses and trains can be cheap and helpful for short distance travel. Air travel can be expensive. Prefer a 21-day advance booking of flight to get 45–50% low rate of the airfare. But there are a very few seats available during this time and a lot of people travel during the holiday season which further limits this option. Other than this, discount on online flight booking may be available in *The New Physician* section of the AAMC (Association of American Medical Colleges), AMSA (American Medical Student Association) and other similar groups. Some applicants also take yearlong membership cards of a particular airline during this time, to avail discounts and maximum benefits. One thing that may help your travel is to know that many nationality licenses are accepted in the United States for driving; few states require international permit along with the license. Please verify if your country license is valid here. If so,

Travel Preparation

In this section we would like to share a few tips for safe air travel:

• Try to arrive your destination at least a day prior to the scheduled pre-interview dinner. This would give a chance to explore the city where you and your family plan to stay for the next 3–4 years.
• The weather conditions during this season are unpredictable, so be prepared to expect flight delays, last moment cancelation and unfavorable accommodations. Prefer flights with moderate layover time in order to compensate for any flight delays.
• Prefer to take an early morning flight or a late-night flight. There are fewer delays in these flights and are usually less expensive.

- Keep all your documents including photo identification, tickets, and interview documents along with airline customer care number or toll-free number in hand.
- Try to avoid cold sandwiches or salads and prefer to eat freshly cooked food or light meals while travelling to avoid any gastro-intestinal issues. Always carry bottled water and a snack in your handbag. Most airlines do not offer meals on board.
- Be aware of the time zone! Make sure to set your watches according to the time zone you are in.
- Familiarize yourself beforehand with the city and the area information to ensure safe travels.
- Just in case you are more prone to falling ill, keep in hand the travel medications like over the counter pain medications, medications for nausea vomiting, medication for gastrointestinal infections or urinary tract infections.
- Carry a travel pillow and eyeshade for comfortable travel. Remember you want to be fresh for the interview day!
- Make sure to check the weather conditions beforehand for snow storms and rains and your winter clothing accordingly.

Housing

Lodging during the interview season can be another expensive issue. Some applicants try to cover up the cost by staying with friends and family in that area. But make sure to check beforehand the distance and estimate the time required to reach the hospital on interview day. Cheap housing can be made available by American Medical Association Alliance along with the American Medical Student Section and American Resident/Fellow Section. These associations run Physician-In-Training Host Program, to help the applicants find cheap housing during the interview season. More information can be made available on their website, and it is advisable to contact the host and confirm the booking at least 2 weeks prior to the expected stays.

The American Medical Women Association also run the similar services to provide cheap housing, but because of the busy interview season, it is advisable to confirm the bookings at least 30 days prior to the expected stays, as they work on first come first served basis.

Cheap lodging is also available through Airbnb® (bed and breakfast) website. But make sure to check the safety of the area beforehand and also confirm the distance of commute to the hospital during the interview day.

Lastly, contact the residency program coordinator where you are interviewing, and they can provide you with discount coupons and convenient options of safe and inexpensive stay near the hospital area.

Conclusion

Travelling and lodging during the interview season can be cumbersome and expensive. But proper planning and coordination beforehand can make your stay comfortable and manage the expenses. Also, this is a good time to explore a new city so make sure you take out some time to relax and venture exciting places and nearby areas and be fresh and prepared for the interview day!

Chapter 20
How Do I Ace Interviews?

Harleen Kaur and Sachin M. Bhagavan

Be so good, they can't ignore you

Introduction

Most residency interviews like any other job interviews are time for self-promotion. It is your best chance to sell yourself with your best attributes in your application and personality to the interviewer. The key to ace an interview is good rehearsal and preparation for the interview. Always practice your interview questions and go well prepared for an interview. Remember you have just 15–20 minutes to impress each faculty!

H. Kaur (✉)
Adesh Institute of Medical Sciences and Research, Bathinda, India

Department of Neurology, University of Missouri, Columbia, MO, USA
e-mail: kaurha@health.missouri.edu

S. M. Bhagavan
Department of Neurology, University of Missouri, Columbia, MO, USA

© Springer Nature Switzerland AG 2020   125
R. Govindarajan et al. (eds.), *International Medical Graduate and the United States Medical Residency Application*,
https://doi.org/10.1007/978-3-030-31045-5_20

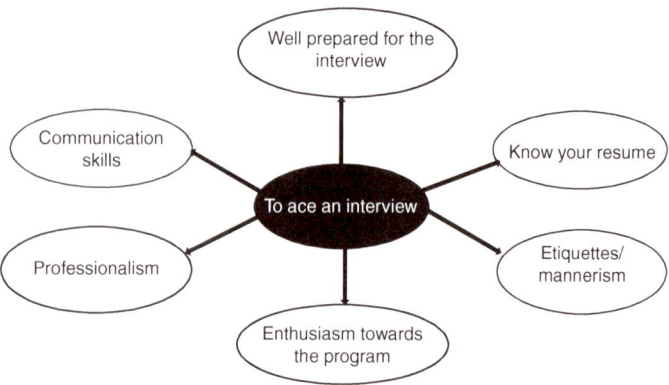

FIGURE 20.1 Shows how to ace an interview

This chapter aims to highlight minute details on how to polish your interview skills and ace your interview. Figure 20.1 shows how to ace an interview in a glance.

Pre-interview Dinner

Pre-interview dinner is a semi-formal social gathering a day prior to the interview day, where the applicants get a chance to meet the residents and other applicants. Pre-interview dinner is a good time to make a nice impression on the residents. Since it is a semi-formal gathering so always be responsive in a friendly and polite way. Don't begin the dinner with the list of questions you have for the program, but start a conversation and then gradually tuck in questions you have about the program. Always begin the conversation as "How was your day?" and "The place looks really nice!"

Avoid sitting quietly during the dinner or just eating the food. Avoid consuming alcoholic beverages. Always be courteous and offer residents first. This is your best chance to interact with the residents, show them enthusiasm about the program and the city area. We will discuss the questions that should be asked to the residents separately later in this chapter. Not all the programs offering interview offer a pre-interview dinner. So if offered, make the most of it to know about the program.

Attire for this event has been discussed above in the previous chapters.

Interview

Be well prepared for the interview. Rehearse your questions and answers well before the interview day. It is important that the applicant should be aware of his/her strengths and present their best qualities on the interview day. The applicants should know what they are looking for in a program and seize every opportunity to know more about the residency program. Figure 20.1 highlights the tips to ace a residency interview.

Always prefer to ask simple straightforward open-ended questions. It is very important to ask the right questions to the right people. Further, in the chapter we will talk about the appropriate questions to be asked the program director, the faculty and residents.

Etiquettes

During the interview, you should always be polite, respectful, and professional toward other applicants, program coordinators, faculty members, and everyone else you meet in the hospital. Always wear a smile and carry a positive attitude. Don't be shy or hesitant; remember it is your chance to know the program as well. The first impression counts a lot, so, you should be dressed professionally and carry a positive body language appropriate for the interview. Always remember you interviewer's name and greet him/her with a firm handshake. Throughout the interview carry a positive attitude and show enthusiasm in the program.

During the lunch time, show good table manners. Don't overeat or put too much in your plate. Avoid food items that have higher chances of spilling over like soups or salads. Always use a fork and knife and eat in small bites. It is better to practice eating etiquettes beforehand if you are not used to using a fork and a knife. Lunch time is the time to interact with the residents and other faculty members; hence it is important to focus more on that than the food.

After the interview ends, there will be tour of the hospital. There is one person (usually a resident) who gives the tour to about 10–15 applicants (approximate number of applicants called on an interview day). Don't follow the crowd or stand at the back, show great enthusiasm in the tour. Remember, actual residency would be more hectic and tiring than an interview day! If you show that you are exhausted or disinterested then how can the program believe that you can pull through residency!! Be inquisitive about the different areas you want to explore like the on-call room, the intensive care unit, emergency room, inpatient services, procedure rooms, simulation labs. At the end of the day, make sure to be thankful to the program coordinators for their assistance throughout the day!

One thing you should always keep in mind on your interview day is that you are selected for interview because the program finds you are as capable as the other candidates. Do not get intimidated by other candidates and do not in any way think that you are inferior to them. At times during interview, there will be moments which won't go as you thought; those moments should not define your entire day! Instead pick yourself up and be in high spirits throughout the day.

Kinds of Interviews

One on one

It is usually the most common type. Typically you will be interviewed by one of the faculty members in his/her office and can last for 15–20 min. Some programs are very strict about their interaction time with the candidates and they keep a timer, but many programs follow informal sense of time and may go up to 30 min. The interview is generally informal and would pertain questions on your CV, personality. Basically they are trying to find out whether you would be a fit to their program and trying to see your personality that they should be aware of before considering you in their rank list. The most important aspect during such interview is to answer honestly and be yourself. If you do not know the answer, you can say "I do not know," but at the same time, be open that you would be glad to get back with an answer to him/her through email if that's appropriate. If you feel your thoughts contradict with that of the interviewer, it is fine to politely say that you do not agree because of this reason, but do not reply rudely or get into an argument with the interviewer. If he/she is persistently enforcing the fact then politely diffuse the situation by acknowledging his/her thoughts. Usually medical knowledge is not evaluated as that is evident by your step scores and LOR.

Panel interview

You might face this type of interview although less frequently. In this type there will be two or more faculty members along with residents of the program. This might look intimidating, but the key to ace such interview is to remain yourself and be alert as you might face two or more questions simultaneously. Calmly answer one after another and make eye contact with all the members present which projects you as a confident applicant.

Group interview

This type of interview is very rare and is the least effective form of interview. In this type, one or more faculty members interview with a group of applicants simultaneously. This is usually to save time. This is the least effective form as there is no effective two-way communication, i.e. you are not able to know about the program and the faculty members and similarly they are not able to know you personally.

Situational type

You may face such type of interview occasionally. In this type, faculty member interviews a group of applicants, usually three to four. You would be given a situation where you are supposed to discuss it with other applicants and all come up with a unified solution in a stipulated time. Usually the interviewer doesn't interrupt and is a mere observer in this scenario. This would test your ability to communicate effectively among peers and your convincing ability but at the same time whether you have the ability to listen to other members patiently and avoid having an argument.

Frequent Questions Asked to the Faculty

Always prefer to ask open-ended questions. Do not go into the details of the subject or educational matter. At the end of the interview the faculty always gives you time to ask the questions. Make sure to ask right questions to the faculty. This will ensure your interest in the residency program. Just in case no questions come to your mind during the interview, then you can tell them as, "*Most of the questions I had were answered by the presentation in the morning and the residents in the pre-interview dinner*."

Always start the interview in a polite note by sharing pleasantries and being thankful for the interview invitation. Most residency interviews explain the structure, strength and history of the program in their oral presentations on the morning of the interview day. Make sure you don't repeat the questions that were addressed in the morning presentation.

- It is always good to ask about the faculty-resident relationship or any mentor/advisor system in residency program.

- The applicants can also inquire about the non-clinical or administrative responsibilities of the residents during the tenure.
- If you are interested in research and want to pursue research during residency, then you can ask the faculty about the same. Make sure you know thoroughly about your research background and what type of research you want to pursue before addressing it. You can also inquire if the program encourages to present research work at annual conferences and if there is any funding available for the same.
- Similarly, if you have a specific interest in a fellowship program, try to connect with the faculty member in the similar fellowship for better guidance. You can also inquire about the programs elective policies so that you can be more involved in your area of interest.
- Applicants can also inquire about the resident evaluation techniques used in the program. This type of question is usually addressed to the program director or chair of the department. Evaluation is helpful in learning and improving into a better physician.
- Applicants can also inquire about any recent changes/advances in the program if they were not mentioned earlier.

Frequent Questions Asked to the Residents

Applicants will get an opportunity to ask the questions to the residents during the pre-interview dinner or during the lunch. As aforementioned both are semi-formal occasions to discuss about the program, so the applicants should maintain decent etiquettes and professionalism at the same time.

- Always begin by asking about the city and the area around the hospital. This type of question is useful in semiformal situations and will give an idea about the place you want to settle in for the next 3–4 years.

- You can enquire about the strengths of the program from the resident point of view. In some questions the opinion of the resident and the faculty both matters. In such situations you can ask the faculty members as "Dr. J, I asked the residents about this (your question) in the pre-interview dinner but I would also like to have your opinion on the same." This is a good chance to show your communication skills and how much you are interested in the program.

- The applicants can also inquire about the resident faculty relationship. You can also inquire if the attending are available on the nights or on weekends and how frequently can you contact them. Also, enquire about the chief resident and their potential role in the program.

- It is good to know about the didactic session in the program. Knowledge and education are equally important in the residency training. The applicant should know how much didactics is offered during a week. Also, try to enquire if you can get a chance to attend didactic session or noon conference or grand rounds during the interview day.

- Try to know about the on-call schedule and the night float system in the program. This will give you an idea how the program distributes their services and call schedules.

- Also try to connect with the residents in an informal way, by asking them what places do they like the most in the city and where do they like to socialize. Or if you have a family and kids, you can also enquire about the housing options and schooling in the city.

Handling Inappropriate/Illegal Questions

There are certain questions which are not ethical or legal to be asked. But yet, you never know. You might come across some interview where you are asked those questions. NRMP has made it very clear not to ask such questions. The interviewer cannot ask you:

- How many programs you have applied?
- How many interviews have you got?

- Any particular geographical locations where you have got most of the interviews?
- How would you rank the programs and where will you rank this program?
- Whether you have plans of having children, if so when?
- Questions about your age, race, ethnicity, religious practices, sexual orientation

If you encounter such questions and you are comfortable answering them, you are most welcome to do so. But if you are uncomfortable about it, then you can politely try to ask the interviewer about the relevance of the question to the residency. This gives an opportunity for the interviewer to go back on it and hence diffuse the situation; do not automatically think that the interviewer has some illegal or discriminatory intent. Many a times, these questions are innocent and are an attempt to get to know you personally. Even after trying politely, you encounter such questions, you can humbly refuse to answer them, or walk out. Remember, doing this would jeopardize your interview and may cost you a match at that program. So think very carefully before taking such drastic steps.

Things to Avoid During an Interview

As important it is to self-promote and present your best attributes forward, keep in mind that you should not sound too arrogant or judgmental during the interview as well. The following are the list of things that applicants should avoid during an interview:

- Do not chew gums, bite nails or smoke during an interview. Chewing gum or blowing bubbles is highly inappropriate and not recommended during an interview. Biting nails is a sign of nervousness and you should not make it obvious by doing that. Smoking during the intervals in the interview is inappropriate and discouraged. Go through the smoking policy of the hospital just in case it is hard for you to resist it. Also, avoid alcohol beverages during the pre-interview dinner.

- Do not talk about other programs and faculty where you have already interviewed or going for an interview. This shows discouragement to the program you are interviewing at.
- Do not ask about the salary, meal plan, vacations and other benefits gained during residency. Most of the residency program has this information available on their website. Such type of questions may sound inappropriate and portray a negative attitude during the interview.
- Do not ask about the moon lighting rules to the residents or faculty. Most residency program discourages moonlighting. Such type of questions may show lack of commitment toward the program.

Conclusion

Interviews can be stressful, but the key to ace the interview is by showing positive attitude and enthusiasm toward the program. Know your resume thoroughly and be well prepared. Always try to be genuine, humble, and polite during the interviews; you never know this program can be your home for the next 3–4 years!

Chapter 21
I Am Done with My Interviews, What Should I Do Now?

Harleen Kaur

> *Success seems to be largely a matter of hanging on, after others have let go ~Anonymous*

Introduction

Once you are done with the interview, don't be relaxed that it is over. You still have time to outshine over other applicants with one last effort. Post-interview follow-up is important for the applicants to emphasize their interest in the program and to maximize their chances of matching to the desired program.

This chapter will highlight important things to keep in consideration after the interview is over.

H. Kaur (✉)
Adesh Institute of Medical Sciences and Research, Bathinda, India

Department of Neurology, University of Missouri, Columbia, MO, USA
e-mail: kaurha@health.missouri.edu

© Springer Nature Switzerland AG 2020   135
R. Govindarajan et al. (eds.), *International Medical Graduate and the United States Medical Residency Application*,
https://doi.org/10.1007/978-3-030-31045-5_21

Evaluate the Program

Most applicants have a lot of interviews, which makes it hard at the end to remember the specifications of each program. Hence it is important to make notes of the program, highlighting the specific details that you liked about the program. This will help you to analyze the strength of the program and rank them accordingly. A program evaluation should be based on the applicant's individual discretion; however there are a few points every applicant should analyze while evaluating the program:

- Clinical experience
- Work environment
- Resident job satisfaction and inter resident relationship
- Stable faculty and resident-faculty interaction
- Didactics sessions
- Research opportunities
- Fellowship opportunities
- Location of the training program and the type of population served

Major factors to keep in mind during evaluation of the program are further listed in the Fig. 21.1.

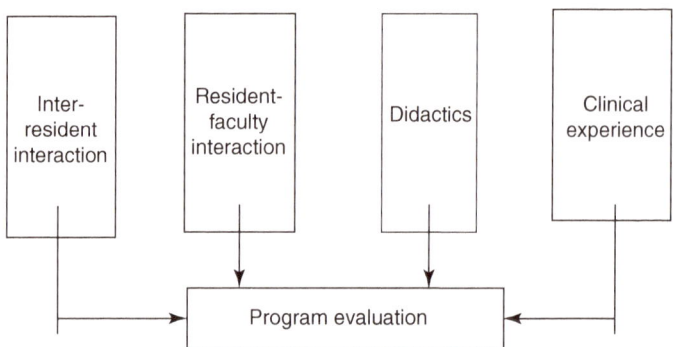

FIGURE 21.1 Shows key factors to consider while evaluating the program

Thank You Correspondence Mails

Writing "thank you" emails or letters is an effective way to stand out among other applicants. Make sure to send the "thank you" emails within 24 hours of the interview. "Thank you" emails are a good way to express your gratitude and enthusiasm toward the residency training program. Applicants can get the email address of the program directors and all other faculty that they interviewed with, through the program website or the program brochure given to them during the interview day. If it is not made available to you make sure to ask the program coordinators regarding the same. Try to write personalized thank you emails, highlighting a mutual interest or any interesting topic you discussed during the interview. The 'thank you' emails should be simple and brief focusing on your interview experience. These emails should be addressed separately to every faculty member including the program coordinator. Figure 21.2 shows a sample "thank you" email to the program director. Some applicants prefer writing personalized letter or post thank you cards to the program. This is

Letter Format

Dear Dr……

Greetings

First paragraph: Thank them for inviting you to the interview on concerned date. Write about your interview experience in 2-3 lines.

Second Paragraph: Highlight any relevant topic you discussed with them

Third paragraph: Show enthusiasm about the program

Always make sure to let the program director know that the program coordinators were very helpful and the day was very well managed by them.

End the letter with positive affirmations regarding your opinions about the program.

Best Regards,

[Your name]

AAMC ID

FIGURE 21.2 Shows draft of thank-you emails addressed to the program after the interview

also a good approach but may turn to be a bit expensive and time consuming. Emails are a convenient and faster way to send personalized messages to the residency training program expressing your motive. It totally depends on the applicant's discretion whether to choose postal cards or emails; however most applicants prefer emails over postal cards.

Follow-Up with the Program

The applicants can keep in touch with the program coordinators during the interview season through emails. You can email the program directors or concerned faculty regarding any updates in your resume like addition of new scores or latest publications. Make sure not to send repeated emails or too many emails to the program coordinators or the program directors. Also, telephone correspondence to the program directors is not appreciated at all. We all know this is a busy time of the year for them and it is important to keep their time into consideration.

Interview season commence during the holiday season which is time for Christmas and New Year's Eve. You can use this time to send season's greetings emails to the program coordinator. If you happen to revisit the town again make sure to visit the program. This will show your persistent interest in the program.

Following up with the program should be in a very professional way highlighting your pure motive and enthusiasm toward the program. This is your last but important effort to express interest in the program, and it is all worth it at the end!

Part III
Post-interview

Chapter 22
I Matched into Prelim Program, What Should I Do Now?

Sorabh Datta

Only I can change my life, no one can do it for me

First, we will discuss what prelim is. I came across it many times when applicants applying for the residency are confused between categorical and prelim positions. The preliminary year is 1 year of training which allows residents to have training prior and help them in decision-making for advanced specialty program [1]. Prelim training includes rotations in internal medicine and surgery, and they are similar to the categorical internal medicine or surgery training interns go through; also few advance programs have specific rotations for meeting their specialty requirements [2]. Few specialties that need prelim year are:

- Anesthesiology
- Dermatology
- Neurology
- Ophthalmology
- Physical Medicine and Rehabilitation
- Radiology
- Radiation Oncology

S. Datta (✉)
Pravara Institute of Medical Sciences, Ahmednagar, India

© Springer Nature Switzerland AG 2020
R. Govindarajan et al. (eds.), *International Medical Graduate and the United States Medical Residency Application*,
https://doi.org/10.1007/978-3-030-31045-5_22

Preliminary positions are planned for the applicants who are seeking 1 or 2 years of clinical experience as a prerequisite for getting into their choice of advanced programs. Internal medicine, surgery, and some transitional programs offer prelim positions. Many applicants confuse these positions just for getting into the residency as an entry point for completing the full residency in either internal medicine or surgery. These positions were never meant for such things. Instead, international medical graduates (IMGs) should plan well before applying for these prelim positions. Figures 22.1 and 22.2 shows the number of IMGs matched to a prelim position as compared to US graduates in Internal Medicine and Surgery, respectively, in 2018.

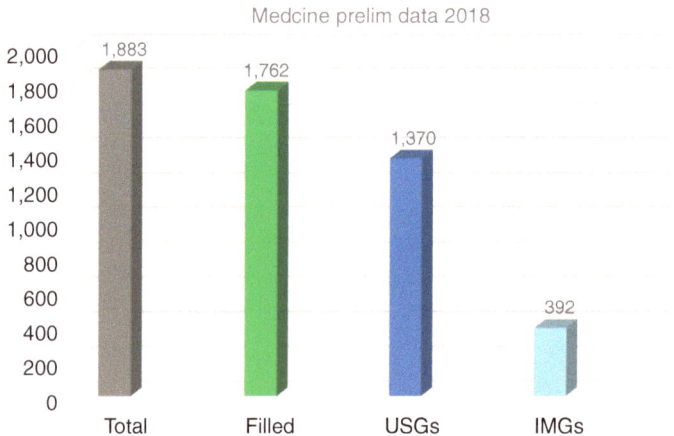

FIGURE 22.1 According to the Results and Data 2018 Main Residency Match, 1883 prelim positions were offered in the internal medicine, out of which 1762 positions were filled among which 392 were IMGs as compared to 1370 US allopathic seniors

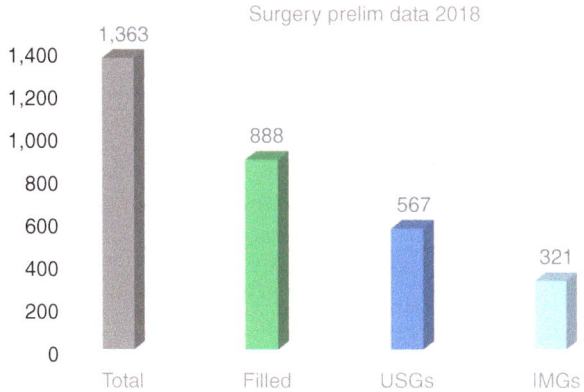

FIGURE 22.2 In surgery, preliminary, 1363 positions were offered and out of which 888 positions were filled. IMGs constitute 321 of those positions as compared to 567 US allopathic seniors [3]

Now the Question Is, Once You Matched into Prelim Year, What's Next?

Well, firstly we have to understand the three different scenarios, either of which we might encounter on the match day.

1. *You got matched*: Time to celebrate!
2. *You remain unmatched*: Time to prepare yourself for the National Resident Matching Program (NRMP) Supplemental Offer and Acceptance Program (SOAP).
3. *You are partially matched*: You matched into the preliminary position but not matched into an advanced position. In this scenario, you are eligible for participating in the SOAP, for getting advanced positions. The entire SOAP process is done in eight rounds, and the candidate has 2 hours to respond for the each match offer. Through SOAP candidate may receive multiple offers.

If You Are Unable to Find Any Advanced Positions in SOAP, Then What?

Well, in this case scenario you have the following options:

- Search for the new advanced positions that got accredited after the SOAP process (the connection with the new program will go out of the NRMP match).
- Search for certain advance positions which remained unfilled due to a resident which decides not to pursue the advanced position.
- You can reapply for the next year categorical position. After you finish 1 year of internship, you have to apply again in matching season for your choice subspecialty.

Let's take an example where an applicant pursuing neurology residency got matched into prelim medicine in the program with preliminary and advance positions. The preliminary interns work side-by-side with other internal medicine categorical residents, rotate through the same hospitals, and are taught by the same faculty. After the intern year in internal medicine, you can start as a PGY2 in the neurology.

There is a rare possibility that you won't end up matching after prelim year, but such cases are uncommon. But in the end, something is better than nothing so always grab the opportunity of prelim position you got and take the most out of it, ultimately preparing yourself for the future.

References

1. Figuring Out the Transitional, Preliminary, and Categorical Year for Residency Application | Doctors in Training. https://www.doctorsintraining.com/blog/figuring-out-the-transitional-preliminary-and-categorical-year-for-residency-application/. Accessed 10 Jan 2019.

2. ACGME Specialties Requiring a Preliminary Year. http://www.acgme.org/Portals/0/PFAssets/ProgramResources/PGY1Requirements.pdf?ver=2017-09-08-114529-173. Accessed 10 Jan 2019.
3. Results and Data 2018 Main Residency Match®. 2018. www.nrmp.org. Accessed 10 Jan 2019.

Chapter 23
I Matched into Advanced Program, What Should I Do Now?

Shanan Mahal

> *Go after your dreams, no matter how unattainable others think it is*

Before we answer this question, let us understand the term advanced programs. Well, these are the programs which start in the PGY-2 year after completing a 1-year prerequisite training, and preliminary programs are those 1-year training programs which begin in the PGY-1 year and provide the necessary prerequisite training for advanced programs. In my previous chapter, I explained to you what happens when you are matched into the preliminary program. So applicants who apply for the advanced programs also apply for the preliminary year simultaneously, or they do it after completing the preliminary year.

When you are searching for a preliminary position on FRIEDA (Fellowship and Residency Electronic Interactive Database), you can also look up for advance positions and nearly all participates in the NRMP (National Resident Matching Program). But most of the

S. Mahal (✉)
Southern Medical University, Guangzhou, China

Department of Internal Medicine, University of Arkansas for Medical Sciences-Baptist Health, North Little Rock, AR, USA

© Springer Nature Switzerland AG 2020   147
R. Govindarajan et al. (eds.), *International Medical Graduate and the United States Medical Residency Application*,
https://doi.org/10.1007/978-3-030-31045-5_23

specialties use separate matches in such cases you need to have done your complete homework to get into those positions. Candidates can also go for joint advance-preliminary tracks, by the NRMP in which you get to apply and rank both positions at the same time. This makes sure applicant who matched in advance gets into the prelim position; it also helps in continuing in the same program till the end if ranked both spots at the same program. For this need an applicant has to create a joint A/P program [1]. Tables 23.1 and 23.2 show the number of advanced positions filled by IMG as compared to USG [2].

TABLE 23.1 PGY-2 positions as per 2018 USG (US graduates) and IMGs include both US IMG and non-US IMG

Specialty	Positions	Total filled	USGs	IMGs
Anesthesiology	447	442	342	100
Child neurology	8	7	4	3
Dermatology	426	420	400	20
Interventional radiology	98	98	96	2
Neurodevelopment disabilities	4	2	2	0
Neurology	287	283	225	58
Nuclear medicine	3	3	0	3
Physical medicine and rehab	281	281	258	23
Radiation oncology	177	172	169	3
Radiology-diagnostic	944	939	837	102
Radiology-nuclear medicine	3	3	2	1
Total PGY-2	2678	2650	2335	315

TABLE 23.2 Physician (R) positions as per 2018 are PGY-2 positions starting in the year of match that are reserved for applicants who have prior graduate medical education (GME)

Specialty	Positions	Total filled	USGs	IMGs
Anesthesiology	140	120	92	28
Child neurology	26	12	7	5
Dermatology	21	20	20	0
Interventional radiology	3	3	2	1
Neurodevelopment disabilities	7	2	2	0
Neurology	20	18	3	15
Nuclear medicine	2	1	1	0
Physical medicine and rehab	7	7	6	1
Radiation oncology	1	1	0	1
Radiology-diagnostic	30	25	19	6
Total physician (R)	257	209	152	57

Physician (R) positions are not available for senior medical students

So This Raises Another Question; What If I Match in the Advance Program but Not in Preliminary?

Now, this is something regrettable because if you don't match in the preliminary program, you will also lose your advance program position. Technically in this scenario, you will be considered as unmatched here. But don't lose hope; contact the program where you matched in advance and let them know you couldn't get into the preliminary program. In such situation, if your advance program has prelim year position unfilled they can squeeze you in. If not, they can contact other programs to help you get into the prelim position. On your part keep trying for the availability of the prelim positions at:

- www.residentswap.com
- www.inforesidency.com
- www.aamc.org/findaresident

These websites help year-around applicants looking for advance positions (PGY-2), prelim year positions (PGY-1), transfer to different program or switching specialty. Start with home institution and contact every possible place. As you matched in advance, that makes you a more desirable applicant.

Once you have matched in the advanced position, you continue your residency till the end. Therefore it's essential to have a plan and better understanding of how preliminary and advanced positions are allotted so that you can be stress-free when switching between two.

References

1. Joint Advanced-Preliminary Tracks – The Match, National Resident Matching Program. http://www.nrmp.org/joint-advanced-preliminary-tracks/. Accessed 12 Jan 2019.
2. Creating a Joint Advanced/Preliminary (A/P) Arrangement Main Residency Match. https://mk0nrmpcikgb8jxyd19h.kinstacdn.com/wp-content/uploads/2017/09/Create_Joint_AP-MRM-IOIAPD.pdf. Accessed 12 Jan 2019.

Chapter 24
I Didn't Match, How Do I Scramble?

Lakshmi P. Digala

> *Every person who prepares is one less person who panics in crisis.*

What's SOAP?

On the Monday of the match week, an applicant will know if he/she got matched or not. If not, do not lose hope; this is when an applicant automatically get eligibility for SOAP (Supplemental Offer and Acceptance Program). SOAP replaced the post-match scramble by NRMP in 2012. Programs with unfilled positions interview eligible applicants and create preference lists in the NRMP Registration, Ranking, and Results—R3 system and offer positions to applicants in the order of the program's preference through a series of offer rounds. However, it seems a daunting task and confusing for the first time. Henceforth, we describe the eligibility, steps of applying, what to prepare, and expect through the SOAP process, and so forth below.

- *SOAP Eligibility*
- The Friday before the match week, all applicants get an email which states that they are eligible for SOAP

L. P. Digala (✉)
University of Missouri, Columbia, MO, USA

© Springer Nature Switzerland AG 2020
R. Govindarajan et al. (eds.), *International Medical Graduate and the United States Medical Residency Application*,
https://doi.org/10.1007/978-3-030-31045-5_24

irrespective of the match outcome. All applicants, irrespective of their match status, get this email conventionally. Once an applicant is eligible and participating in SOAP, he/she must be within the contract of not contacting the programs directly during the entire process.

All applicants with the following criteria are SOAP eligible:

1. Who are either unmatched or partially matched?
   (Partially matched are those who secured Preliminary PGY1 position and no advance position or who matched into PGY2 advanced position without PGY1 position).
2. Who are eligible to enter graduate medical education by July 1st of that match year.
3. Registered for the main match.

According to 2018 NRMP data [1],

- 13,176 applicants were SOAP eligible.
- 464 out of 525 unfilled programs participated in SOAP, offering 1171 positions.
- 54.7% positions were PGY-1 only. Table 24.1 describes the number of positions available based on specialties.
- 1644 offers were sent to applicants: 1055 were accepted, 542 rejected, and 47 expired.

TABLE 24.1 SOAP positions available according to 2018 NRMP data

Programs participated in SOAP	Number of positions
Prelim surgery	462
Prelim medicine	99
Prelim OB&Gyn	10
Prelim pediatrics	5
Internal medicine	173
Family medicine	117
Pediatrics	59
Anesthesiology	48

- Of those accepted, 55.1% were US seniors, 20% Osteopathic students/graduates, and 20.3% International medical graduates.
- In conclusion, 90.1% (1055 of 1171) of SOAP positions had been filled.

- *SOAP Timeline of Events*

- Some serious thought should be given into the risk of not matching at least few weeks prior to match week, so that you can put some effort on the preparation for the SOAP. Applications documents should be well prepared in advance, which includes if any new letters are being uploaded, Am I still applying to same specialty? If not, new personal statement must be got ready. Herein, we discuss in detail the process of the rounds offered in the SOAP program.

Monday of Match Week

- At 11 am Eastern Standard Time (EST), programs and applicants learn about the match outcome.
- As mentioned above, unmatched or partially matched applicants will get access to the unfilled programs.
- Programs can view an applicant SOAP application only after 3 pm EST, so he/she has time only until 3 pm to work and submit it.
- The maximum number of programs you can apply is 35, so choose wisely.
- From this point, an applicant must be readily available for the programs that might contact till the end of the SOAP season, which is Thursday of the match week.
- Don't fail to attend the phone call or respond to email in a timely manner. If an applicant cannot be reached, the program moves on to the next applicant.
- Make use of the time by getting to know about the programs you have applied, as that helps to make a good impression in the interview process.

Tuesday of Match Week

By Tuesday 11.30, SOAP preference list is created by programs. Unlike NRMP match where both the applicants and the programs create preference list here only the programs get the choice.

Wednesday of Match Week

Wednesday afternoon is when the applicant starts getting offers. Every applicant who gets an offer has 2 hours to accept or reject it. Once an applicant accept the offer, he/she can no longer participate in SOAP, and it becomes an agreement between you and the program. It is strongly suggested to consider accepting an offer as it comes because once rejected, you are not going to receive an offer from the same program. It is tempting to wait for the better offer, but it is always uncertain. So carefully think before rejecting an offer.

- By noon EST—Applicants begin to get offers in round 1.
- By 2 pm EST—Applicants must accept or reject by 2 pm.
- By 3 pm EST—Applicants begin to get offers for unfilled positions in round 2.
- By 5 pm EST—Applicants must accept or reject by 5 pm.

Thursday of Match Week

Thursday is the last day of SOAP, and the timeline is shown below:

- By 9 am EST—Applicants begin to get offers for unfilled positions round 3.
- By 11 am EST—Applicants must have accepted or rejected by 11 am.
- By noon 12 EST—Applicants begin to get offers for unfilled positions in round 4.

- By 2 pm EST—Applicants must have accepted or rejected by 2 pm.
- By 3 pm EST—Applicants begin to get offers for unfilled positions in round 5.
- By 5 pm EST—Applicants must accept or reject by 5 pm.

When an applicant accepts a residency position, the R3 system creates an automatic rejection for further offers, for which the applicant no longer is eligible. If an offer has not been accepted by applicant, a position may be offered in multiple rounds. As soon as the SOAP ends, list of unfilled programs will be made available in the website. From this point you are free to contact those programs.

Reference

1. www.nrmp.org/wp-content/uploads/2018/04/Main-Match-Result-and-Data-2018.pdf.

Chapter 25
I Matched but Not to the Program of My Top Choice, What Do I Do?

Lakshmi P. Digala

Try to get what you like, like what you get

The central goal of the match process run by an algorithm by the NRMP (National Resident Matching Program) is to match the choices of both applicants and the residency program at its best. Still, that might not be true always, and applicants might end up in the program of not their option. Hunting down for such a compatible position and the transfer is a daunting task, like applying for a new job. Herein, we discuss in detail such scenarios and diverse selections available to address them.

The latest NRMP data in 2018 showed the most significant match rate that has been witnessed ever since 2003. 73.3% of the US seniors matched to one of their top three choices. The graph in Fig. 25.1 shows the match percentage of the individual applicants to their first choice are 36.6%, and the top three choices are more than half, which is 51.5% [1].

According to 2018 match data from the NRMP, for US IMG (international medical graduates) represented in the following (Fig. 25.2), the top five choice specialties in the descending order of matching were:

L. P. Digala (✉)
University of Missouri, Columbia, MO, USA

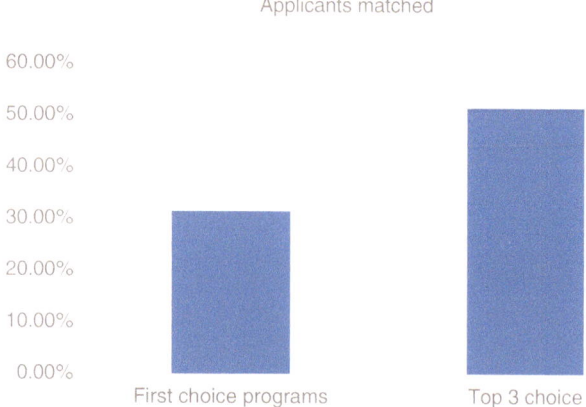

FIGURE 25.1 Graph of individual applicants matched to their program of choice (2018) [1]

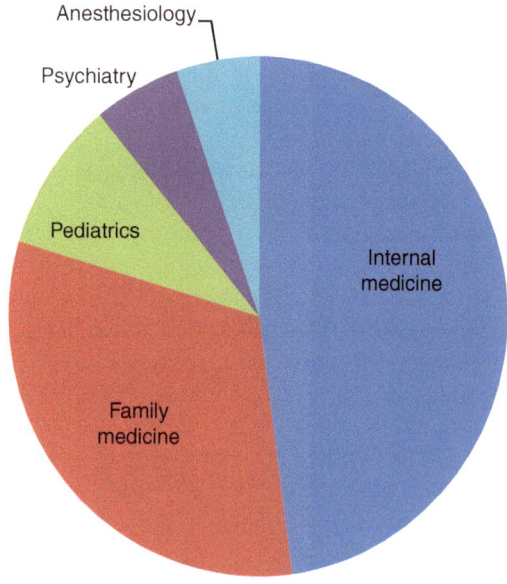

FIGURE 25.2 US-IMG matched data of top 5 specialties—2018 NRMP

- Internal Medicine (1107)
- Family Medicine (735)
- Pediatrics (218)
- Psychiatry (129)
- Anesthesiology (125)

The top five specialties for non-US IMG in the descending order of matching as seen in Fig. 25.3 are:

- Internal Medicine (2076)
- Family Medicine (330)
- Pediatrics (categorical) (315)
- Neurology (192)
- Pathology (185)

According to a study published in JAMA surgery, which surveyed more than 300 residents; the most common reasons

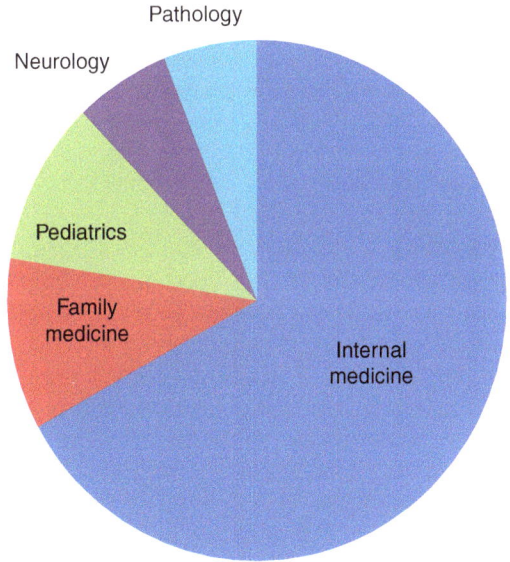

FIGURE 25.3 Non US-IMG matched data of top 5 specialties—2018 NRMP

of a resident to leave the program are sleep deprivation, absence of faculty members, and excessive work hours on rotation. On the contrary, the reasons to stay back in the program are support from the partner, family, other residents, and perception of being rested. Women who are maintaining the balance between motherhood and professional life were the ones more likely to report leaving the residency program [2].

There are various sources where you can find a resident who is interested in the program where you matched, and they are very much interested in swapping their positions. ResidentSwap.org is such a website with vacancy database information where you could find such residents. Here in this website, they post their interest, and even the residency programs as well turn in their interests for any unfilled positions.

Another such source is FRIEDA (Fellowship and Residency Electronic Interactive Database) where one can find aggregate statistics about the open and vacant programs and information about the graduates of programs. This helps you in the research about the program as well. Although switching seems easy if you find open positions before transferring, all the paperwork which the resident did for the current residency position must be redone. The residency program directors from sending and receiving end are the key. But the pressure builds on the residency program director about vacant positions too. Check the program transfer policies ahead of taking the decision about switching [3].

It is of vital importance to be in contact with the program of your choice. The most vital contact could be the program director to the coordinator. Write them to express your interest and stay connected to know if there are any last-minute drops by International medical graduates. Although rare, it is not quite uncommon due to difficulties with the visa issues. This gray period where the incoming residents are supposed to report to join the residency program could be a chance to secure the spot. Periodic communication with the program is vital.

References

1. http://www.nrmp.org/wp-content/uploads/2018/04/Main-Match-Result-and-Data-2018.pdf.
2. https://www.ama-assn.org/residents-students/resident-student-health/top-reasons-residents-leave-their-programs-and-why-they.
3. https://www.ama-assn.org/residents-students/residency/want-switch-residency-programs-5-things-you-should-know.

Chapter 26
I Matched but Not to the Specialty of My Top Choice, What Do I Do?

Shanan Mahal

Always follow your heart. But take your brain with you

Choosing your specialty wisely is very crucial because this decides how your rest of the life will be. For a surgeon in an operating room thinking that he will rot in the operating room for the rest of his life or for a pathologist thinking that he will miss interacting with the patients or for a radiologist missing delivering babies as OB/GYN are various examples of not finding your true love or in simple language not matching in your choice of specialty. This will decrease your productivity and will leave you frustrated for the rest of your life. This is not very uncommon because sometimes while doing a rotation in the medical school, time is not enough to take a decision, or you did not properly think it through while making the decision.

The regret of not matching at your first choice of specialty is common especially when candidates apply in multiple

S. Mahal (✉)
Southern Medical University, Guangzhou, China

Department of Internal Medicine, University of Arkansas for Medical Sciences-Baptist Health, North Little Rock, AR, USA

© Springer Nature Switzerland AG 2020   163
R. Govindarajan et al. (eds.), *International Medical Graduate and the United States Medical Residency Application*,
https://doi.org/10.1007/978-3-030-31045-5_26

specialties. It happens very commonly with those IMGs who have average scores and therefore apply multiple specialties to increase their chances of getting matched. As you saw in the previous chapters, roughly 44% of the IMGs remain unmatched as compared to US allopathic seniors who have a success rate of approximately 94% in the matching [1]. That's why some IMGs apply for multiple specialties to increase their chances of getting matched, and in the end, they end up matching in a specialty which is not their top choice, and they are disappointed.

If you are matched not in the specialty of your choice, don't lose hope. Take this opportunity to gain a year of experience of working as a resident in the residency where you matched and try for the next year again if you think that you won't be able to give your 100% to that particular specialty. The knowledge you will acquire in that 1 year will be helpful in your future career. The goal for you is to give your 100% in this noble profession, anything less than that shows your incompetence towards the program.

Job satisfaction is also essential. This path is not easy, but after 30 or more years of your practice, you won't blame yourself for not trying it. Many residents after they do not match at their choice of specialty in a period of 1 year realize that they don't belong there, have disinterest and feel defeated that can be harmful to their work so share your thoughts with your attending or mentor and let them know you are lacking the interest and want to switch to another specialty. In fact, as per the National Physician Burnout & Depression Report, 2018 physicians reported depression and burnout in their specialty as shown in Fig. 26.1. The rate of depression in the following specialties is shown below in Fig. 26.2.

What will be your next steps if you really think that you did not match into your choice of specialty? In short what you will be doing if you are not happy in your current residency program (Fig. 26.3); they are as follows:

1. Talk to your Program Director and your mentors and let them know what you feel because they can help you best in

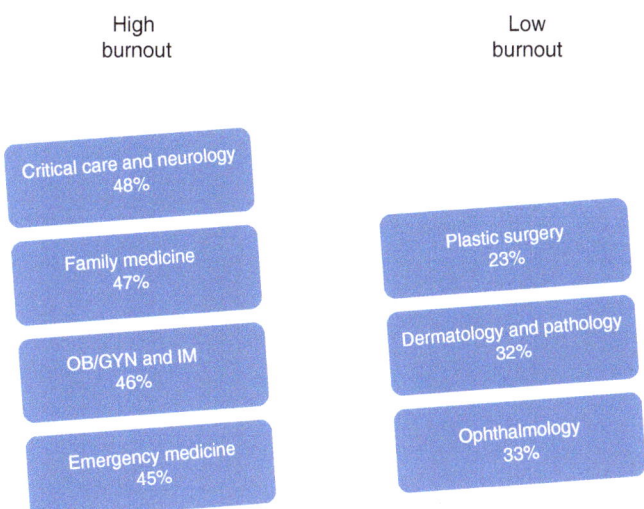

High
burnout

Low
burnout

Critical care and neurology
48%

Family medicine
47%

OB/GYN and IM
46%

Emergency medicine
45%

Plastic surgery
23%

Dermatology and pathology
32%

Ophthalmology
33%

FIGURE 26.1 Comparison between specialties with more stress resulting in more burn out and medical specialties with lower burnout reported [2]

this situation. If your choice of specialty is in the same hospital and that program has a vacancy available, then your Program Director can help with the switching.

2. Keep on looking for the vacancy at your choice of specialties on American Medical Association (AMA) and Resident Swap.

3. Also, remember at starting of your residency, you will be allotted Graduate Medical Education (GME) funding according to your number of years in training. And you will be provided with initial residency period code that stays with you if you are switching to a specialty which is longer than your present training; the teaching hospital will be

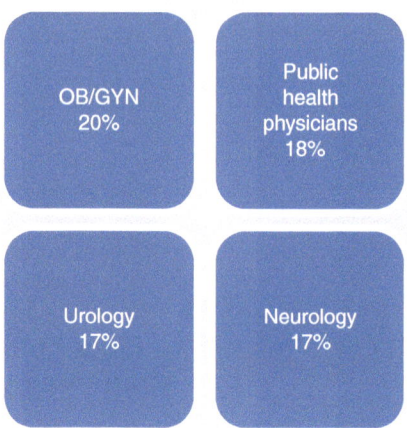

FIGURE 26.2 List of specialties reported with the highest rate of depression [3]

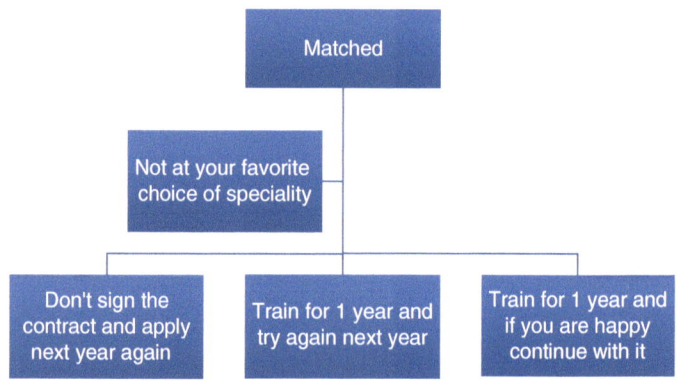

FIGURE 26.3 Shows algorithm for different scenario after matching to non favorite choice of specialty

paid half of your Medicare Direct Graduate Medical Education [4].

4. Once you finish PGY-1, you can apply in PGY-2 or Advanced Programs directly if your choice of specialty needs 1 year of prelim training. Next possibility is you have to repeat PGY-1.

Some residents start liking the specialty after working in it for a year, and consider that life has put them where they are supposed to be. Also for those who are open to everything this route is more comfortable. It is also not uncommon to see candidates matched at their specialty of choice, while training in it for some time they realize that they want something different, and again it will be a big debate in your mind about the time you will give to this specialty vs. your satisfaction. Therefore these decisions are to be taken keeping an open mind because that will not only affect you but also your family and residency programs.

References

1. Main Residency Match Data and Reports – The Match, National Resident Matching Program. http://www.nrmp.org/main-residency-match-data/. Accessed 12 Jan 2019.
2. Physician burnout: It's not you, it's your medical specialty|American Medical Association. https://www.ama-assn.org/residents-students/specialty-profiles/physician-burnout-it-s-not-you-it-s-your-medical-specialty. Accessed 12 Jan 2019.
3. Medscape National Physician Burnout & Depression Report 2018. https://www.medscape.com/slideshow/2018-lifestyle-burnout-depression-6009235#2. Accessed 12 Jan 2019.
4. Medicare Direct Graduate Medical Education (DGME) Payments – Graduate Medical Education (GME) – Government Affairs – AAMC. https://www.aamc.org/advocacy/gme/71152/gme_gme0001.html. Accessed 12 Jan 2019.

Chapter 27
I Matched and I Want to Know What the Next Steps Are?

Shanan Mahal

Hip Hip Hooray! This match day is your day.

You have matched and that is an awesome feeling. Take some time to enjoy this news with your family and friends but get prepared for the other crucial steps you need to take. As in the next few hours and days, you have to do a lot of important things because the real game just begins now!

Consider this, you got the golden match ticket and now you have to board the train which will take you to your ultimate destination which is the residency. You will be firmly attached to this residency program for good amount of time in the coming years. Let's make the checklist of the things you need to be doing after getting matched.

- *Contact the program*: First, reach to your program by an email and phone contact especially with your program coordinator and thank them for this opportunity. Tell your program that how happy you are to be matched in their program and how excited you are to start your residency.

S. Mahal (✉)
Southern Medical University, Guangzhou, China

Department of Internal Medicine, University of Arkansas for Medical Sciences-Baptist Health, North Little Rock, AR, USA

© Springer Nature Switzerland AG 2020 169
R. Govindarajan et al. (eds.), *International Medical Graduate and the United States Medical Residency Application*,
https://doi.org/10.1007/978-3-030-31045-5_27

Make them feel special as they will make you feel special in your residency. Do remember! This will be your new family away from home, and you need everyone's support for getting the best out of your residency. Make a short thank you call to the program director as well for thanking him for this excellent opportunity. This will be the first positive thing in the direction of your employer-employee relationship. Ask for any additional paperwork you need to send them [1].

- *Signing the contract with your residency program*: The program will send you the contract to sign with them, which will have all the information you will be needing, like:
    - Length of the residency program
    - Your responsibilities in the program
    - Duty hours and procedures
    - Salary and other stipends
    - Liability of insurance provided to you
    - Health insurance of you and your family
    - Leave and vacation policies
    - Moonlighting policies
    - Policies regarding misconduct
    - Other benefits available to you

  Go through all the policies and if you have any questions don't hesitate to ask your program director or your residency coordinator and be open about it Make sure that you completely read and understood everything before signing the contract.

- *Thank you note*: Do send the thank you email or letter to your mentor and everyone who supported you by writing the letter of recommendation for you or who has given you the guidance for this program. The bottom line is that you should be thankful to all those people who have contributed to your success. Let them know that you have matched and how vital their role is in your residency success.

- *Visa*: As an IMG, if you require a visa for your residency program, you need to be in touch with your program and work with them on your visa papers because it is a lengthy process. The J1 visa is easier to obtain, and it is sponsored by the Educational Commission for Foreign Medical Graduates (ECFMG) with a maximum of 7 years of duration. Next comes the H1B visa, which is harder to get and sponsored by your residency program with a maximum 6 years of length as per current rules of the permit and it also requires passing of the United States Medical Licensing Examination (USMLE) Step 3 exam. They both are a non-immigrant visa. H-1B allows US employers to temporarily employ foreign workers in specialty occupations, while J-1 visa is issued by the United States to research scholars, professors, and exchange visitors participating in programs that promote cultural exchange, primarily to obtain medical or business training within the United States [2].

- *Talk to the current residents*: They will be your friends, your mentors, and your family. Even they are also excited to see the fresh batch of interns in their programs. This senior, junior bond will be your first test as a team member in your residency program. It's crucial to gel well with the current residents as you have to work with them as a team. Be in touch with them through phone, email or social network. They will guide you in settling down in the new area. They will guide you in moving to the new house, eating places and the most important thing they will guide you is in surviving the hard residency.

- *Housing, Packing and Moving*: Start looking for the rental apartments, always try to find the place which is near to your workplace. This will make your daily commute to your hospital easier especially on the lousy weather day. Also look for transit options near to it. If you have your own vehicle, then look for places which provide safe parking for your vehicle [3, 4]. (More information on this is given in the Chap. 29, what should I pack and not pack).

- *USMLE Step 3*: If you are left with this exam, then this is the best time to complete with it. Once you are cleared with the USMLE Step 3 exam, you will have one less thing to worry about your residency and ultimately you will enjoy your residency more. Many candidates start planning to study for Step 3 before joining the residency as it will also help them brush all the topics and assists them in the start of their internship year. The earlier you start your preparation, it is easier for you to take the exam during your internship year [3, 4].

- *Vacation*: It sounds very nonsense, but trust me it's better to plan your vacation well in advance. The bottom line is advance planning before starting the new journey of your life.

References

1. Starting residency well – residency. https://www.aafp.org/medical-school-residency/residency/start.html. Accessed 12 Jan 2019.
2. Stovner L, Hagen K, Jensen R, et al. The global burden of headache: a documentation of headache prevalence and disability worldwide. Cephalalgia. 2007;27(3):193–210. https://doi.org/10.1111/j.1468-2982.2007.01288.x.
3. So you matched to a residency program–now what?|American Medical Association. https://www.ama-assn.org/residents-students/match/so-you-matched-residency-program-now-what. Accessed 12 Jan 2019.
4. 5 Steps to take after match day. https://www.medscape.com/viewarticle/876536. Accessed 12 Jan 2019.

Chapter 28
I Didn't Match This Year, Should I Apply Again?

Shanan Mahal

> *Be patient, sometimes you have to go through the worst to get the best*

It is depressing to see not getting matched. It takes some time to overcome it and find out the reasons where you lacked. The one significant reason for not matching is the high applicant to positions ratio, and that we can't change, but we still have a lot to improve. Then comes the question "Do I quit?" and, the answer is *NO*. After giving years of hard work in preparing the United States Medical Licensing Examination (USMLE), gaining US clinical experience (USCE) and lot of investment, this all can't be left behind with just one failure.

So, the answer to the question "I didn't match this year, should I apply again?" is *YES*, you should apply again. The moment you hear not matched news you need to find where did you lack and how you can work on it and make your application look better for next year. In this chapter, we will review the conditions which went wrong and how you can improve on them. Reasoning out the possibilities is the most crucial step.

S. Mahal (✉)
Southern Medical University, Guangzhou, China

Department of Internal Medicine, University of Arkansas for Medical Sciences-Baptist Health, North Little Rock, AR, USA

© Springer Nature Switzerland AG 2020   173
R. Govindarajan et al. (eds.), *International Medical Graduate and the United States Medical Residency Application*,
https://doi.org/10.1007/978-3-030-31045-5_28

Reasons for Not Getting Matched

1. *USMLE scores*: The low scores or an attempt in any USMLE exam is something essential when it comes to interviewing, also among one of the weakness that you can't change. But you can still work on other fields for the next year to make them compensate. But this particular thing will be a major filter in most of the program's application filter. Mean score of applicants who matched for each specialty per NRMP data is shown in Table 28.1.

2. *USCE*: When we say USCE it does not just have Letter of Recommendations (LORs) from anywhere, it carries a lot of value, so you need to have a rotation done from a teaching hospital and try to have hands-on clinical experience if possible. Also, make sure you have very good LORs. So, for next year, start working on it especially in the specialty where you are applying. If you are still in medical school, you can apply for a Clinical Elective; if already graduated look for Externship over Observership as it is more valuable because of direct patient care. Externships are harder to get because they are limited in number due to legal restrictions; if you are interested in Observership, you can visit AMA website for the list of programs providing Observership for International Medical Graduates [1].

3. *Research*: This condition varies from program to program, few programs prefer research significantly, and with this, they mean published papers and experience in the lab. It is always better to volunteer for research for a year in teaching hospitals; this helps to improve the application, and it will boost your chances in getting research-oriented programs. Figure 28.1 shows the mean number of research experience and the mean number of abstracts, presentations, and publications required for matching as per NRMP data 2018 [2].

4. *Applying date*: Website of ERAS has clearly mentioned all the deadlines for submission. Visit the website of ERAS timeline which clearly specifies the start date for applying,

TABLE 28.1 Shows mean USMLE step 1 and 2 scores of US IMG and non-US IMG applicants who matched per NRMP data 2018

	US IMG		Non-US IMG	
	Step 1	Step 2	Step 1	Step 2
Anesthesiology	231	237	240	244
Child neurology	–	–	235	242
Dermatology	–	–	238	246
Diagnostic radiology	239	242	241	243
Emergency medicine	232	241	229	234
Family medicine	211	225	220	231
General surgery	237	245	242	249
Internal medicine (IM)	225	234	236	241
IM/pediatrics	224	233	238	240
Neurological surgery	–	–	246	243
Neurology	227	234	236	240
Obstetrics and gynecology	229	238	231	237
Orthopedic surgery	239	245	239	237
Pathology	226	230	230	233
Pediatrics	221	232	230	238
Physical medicine and rehabilitation	226	235	238	242
Plastic surgery	–	–	228	242
Psychiatry	214	227	222	232
Vascular surgery	–	–	243	247

Few data are not shown due to the small sample size

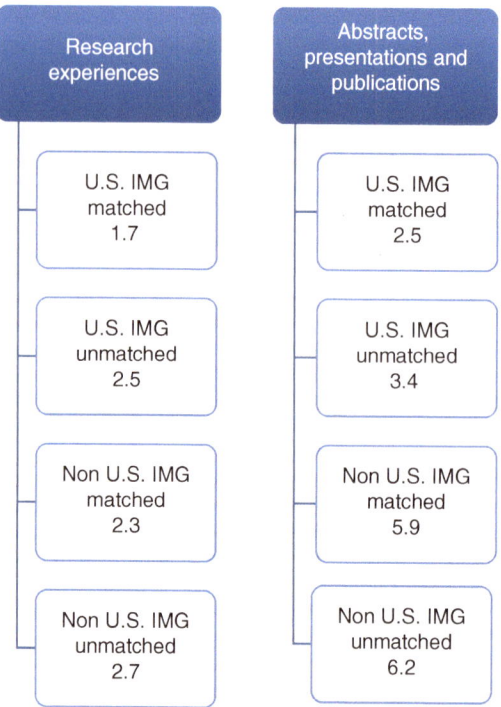

FIGURE 28.1 Provides statistics of all specialties combined NRMP data 2018 for matched vs. not matched IMG

the date the program starts receiving an application, and also when Medical Student Performance Evaluation (MSPE) is released to the residency programs. You can still submit late, but lots of programs already go through the applications in September and start to send the invites by October. Applying late can be harmful so plan properly and get all the paperwork done at the right time [3].

5. *Programs applying*: When you are applying, you have to go broadly in your choice of specialty and do research on the programs before you apply. See the criteria they are looking in for an applicant. If you don't meet the requirements for any program, it can filter out your application which can decrease the number of interviews.

6. *Incomplete application*: This is a mistake which is very often to be made. So be very careful and read thoroughly before submitting the application. Also, write everything correctly because this reflects you as an irresponsible or a lousy applicant and it can harm the invitations. Link to the website is mentioned in the references where you will find the answer to all the question regarding ERAS application [4].

7. *Personal statement*: In this book, previously we have explained the importance of personal statement and how it can be a major factor in getting an interview invite. Mistakes done in the personal statement can negatively harm your application. So, for next year work on it and take time to write it.

8. *Specialty*: It matters a lot in which specialty you are applying based on your scores, your LORs. So, if you are applying to some competitive specialty, you need to have good USCE in it along with their mean scores. So, for your top choice specialty work on gaining useful experience for next year. The Table 28.1 shows the mean score needed for any specialty as per 2018 NRMP data.

9. *Interviews*: We have already mentioned in the book about the number of interviews needed to secure a residency position. Less number can be stressful, but if you work on your interview skills you can still achieve it. Remember, all you require is one position in one residency program! For next year prepare for your interview, because that few minutes in the room can change your life.

10. *Ranking*: Rank order list (ROL) needs to be done smartly, try to rank all the programs, and choose the one where you want to be in and not by how was your interview or what the interviewer said.

Besides working on the above mentioned things in the period of 1 year, you can finish your Step 3 exam which does shoot up the chance of interviews. As per NRMP program director survey 2018 USMLE step 3 score carry 16% citing factor while selecting the applicant for the interview [5]. You can also gain a secondary degree in a year like Master of

Public Health (MPH), Master of Healthcare Administration (MHA) and Master of Business Administration (MBA) which will be a beneficial addition to your application. In the end, it is imperative to use the whole year mindfully to make next year application look stronger for your residency position.

References

1. Observership program listings for international medical graduates|American Medical Association. https://www.ama-assn.org/education/international-medical-education/observership-program-listings-international-medical. Accessed 8 Feb 2019.
2. Charting outcomes in the match: international medical graduates characteristics of international medical graduates who matched to their preferred specialty in the 2018 main residency match 2nd edition. 2018. www.nrmp.org. Accessed 8 Feb 2019.
3. ERAS 2019 Timeline for IMG Residency. https://students-residents.aamc.org/applying-residency/article/eras-timeline-img-residency/. Accessed 8 Feb 2019.
4. Frequently Asked Questions for ERAS Residency Applicants. https://students-residents.aamc.org/applying-residency/faq/faq-eras-residency-applicants/. Accessed 8 Feb 2019.
5. Results of the 2018 NRMP Program Director Survey. 2018. www.nrmp.org. Accessed 7 Feb 2019.

Chapter 29
How to Prepare for a Life in the USA?

Lakshmi P. Digala

The best view comes after the hardest climb

The Big Dream

Being in the USA is a big dream for most of the people in the world. As physicians, we are fortunate to see the largest match season ever in 2018. According to NRMP data, as in Table 29.1, the number of total and filled positions is increasing, giving a positive outlook toward one's matching dream.

Culture in the USA

The USA is an amalgamation of various diverse ethnicities and races, although predominantly populated by white Americans. The incoming resident physicians come from different countries with diverse cultures and upbringing; it is imperative to initially get an insight of various elements. Majority of them include cultural practices, languages, and

L. P. Digala (✉)
University of Missouri, Columbia, MO, USA

179
R. Govindarajan et al. (eds.), *International Medical Graduate and the United States Medical Residency Application*,
https://doi.org/10.1007/978-3-030-31045-5_29

TABLE 29.1 Shows NRMP data about total positions and filled positions as compared to 2017

Residency	Number (2018)	Change from 2017	
Total positions	33,167	↑ 1410	4.40%
Total positions filled	31,899	↑ 1421	4.70%
PGY-1 positions	30,232	↑ 1383	4.80%
PGY-1 positions filled	29,040	↑ 1352	4.90%

other aspects of the USA where you are going to live. This helps to ease the process of acclimatization. Herein we provide an insight into the practice of medicine influenced by various elements of the culture.

Language

Although English is the primary language spoken in the USA, which is the de facto national language, Spanish is the second most common language in the country. Approximately 41 million people of the USA population speak Spanish according to the 2015 census. Figure 29.1 depicts the distribution of languages in the USA.

Language discordance may hinder effective healthcare delivery [1]. Spanish is the second most commonly spoken language next to English. They constitute a significant portion of the patient population in underserved areas. Recent studies reported that people speaking Spanish are less satisfied with the healthcare they receive than their white counterparts. Their satisfaction, which was measured by a physician's friendliness, concern, and ability to make the patient comfortable, was studied. It was reported that they perceive that physicians fail to provide the needed information [2]. Language barrier leading to a lack of explanation of side effects of medication seemed to negatively correlate with the compliance of medication as per a study done in an underserved Hispanic community.

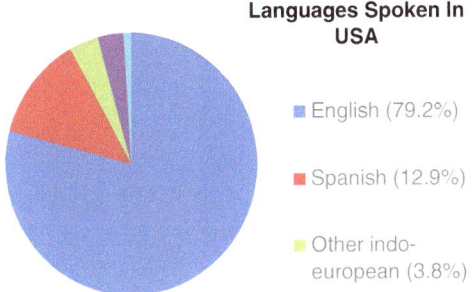

Languages Spoken In USA

- English (79.2%)
- Spanish (12.9%)
- Other indo-european (3.8%)

FIGURE 29.1 Shows different languages spoken in the USA

The interpreters were used to overcome this defect. When an interpreter was used during clinical visits, the patient satisfaction was also reportedly low [3]. While the use of interpreters is a common practice, errors in medical interpretation are quite high, with a mean of 31 per encounter in a study [4]. The errors committed by ad hoc interpreters had potential clinical consequences than hospital interpreters. The most common errors are omission about drug allergies, drug dose, and drug frequency. The remote simultaneous interpretation replaced the traditional proximate consecutive interpretation. There was a lower rate of inaccurately interpreted utterances with remote simultaneous interpretation, and patients preferred this over traditional type.

Religion

The practice of medicine is based on the practice of the principle of the patient's autonomy. Religion and its belief play a significant role in a decision-making capacity, especially with medical treatment options conflicting with their belief system. Table 29.2 describes the distribution of religions in the USA according to the latest survey.

As a healthcare provider, the role of religion as a humanitarian aspect of holistic care and its effectiveness in determining the health level of patients and their family members

TABLE 29.2 Percentage of religions in the USA

Religions in the USA (2016)	% of US population
Christian	69
Catholic	20
Mormon	1
Jehovah's Witness	1
Non-Christian	7
Jewish	2
Muslim	1
Buddhist	1
Hindu	1
Other non-Christian	2

should be well understood. By becoming a resident, one must undertake specific and demanding moral obligations. A resident is bound to fulfill them as part of professionalism. Great doctors are devoted to reaching the goals of medicine for their patients. The rules of autonomy, non-maleficence, beneficence, and justice help the wellness care providers in the decision-making of complex patient care, especially when faced with ethical situations [5].

Insurance

Health Insurance

Among all types of insurances, health insurance plans are one of the essentials for life in the USA. Healthcare delivery is driven by insurance in the USA. It is a form of insurance that provides protection against the cost of medical expenses, and coverage depends on the chosen type of plan an individual. There are several types, that may be privately purchased or funded by the government. Table 29.3 describes several public and private forms of insurances.

TABLE 29.3 Shows healthcare plans in the USA

Government health plans	Private health plans
Medicare	Consumer-driven
Medicaid/State Health Insurance	healthcare
Assistance Program (SHIP)	Flexible Spending
Federal Employee Health Benefits	Account (FSA)
program	Health Savings Account
Military Health System/TRICARE	(HSA)
Veteran's Health administration	Health Reimbursement
Indian Health Service	Account
State Children's Health Insurance	Private Fee for Service
Program (CHIP)	(PFFS)
Prescription Assistance (SPAP)	Managed care (CCP)
Program of all-inclusive care for the	Exclusive Provider
Elderly (PACE)	Organization (EPO)
	Health Maintenance
	Organization (HMO)
	Preferred Provider
	Organization (PPO)

Many of the healthcare reforms have been instituted by the Affordable Care Act of 2010 to promote health coverage. The Health Insurance Portability and Accountability Act— HIPPA (1996) is created to modernize the healthcare flow and stipulate personal identifiable information with health-care systems from theft or fraud. The number of uninsured people has been steadily decreasing and stabilized at 9% of the US population. The major part of private health insurance in the USA is employment-based.

Travel Insurance

This is a type of privately purchased health insurance which is required, especially for those who are applying for B1/B2, H1, J1, and F1 visa. As healthcare cost in the USA is very steep, this will protect you against unexpected events that can cripple you financially. Also, this can be purchased if any of your family or friends are visiting the USA for shorter periods.

Dental Insurance

Dental care is expensive as well unless covered by insurance. Likewise, dental insurance has three options like, private healthcare plans. They are

- Dental Health Maintenance Organization (DHMO)
- Preferred Provider Organization (PPO)
- Indemnity—Fee for service

There are no single best dental plans, and the selection depends on one's family needs. The coverage breaks down into four distinct classes based on care ranging from prevention, basic operations, major procedures, and orthodontics.

Accommodation

Rental Housing

Finding a perfect home to live is no piece of cake in the USA. Various standards are critical in deciding the place. Coping with higher stress and long working hours of residency is not an easy task either. You can find many places for rent on various sites like Craigslist, local community center sites. Always find some handy information from the older residents as they have been through this cycle. Herein we suggest seeing a few factors like neighborhood and access to work. If you have family and children, consider looking right school districts which are carried on the school district website.

Own House

This seems a very laborious process while you begin your residency, and still, it can be made out. However, that place is going to be your home for the next few years based on the speciality you chose. Even if it is your first time, this task is easily performed by learning a few tips. The realtor websites like Trulia, Zillow, and Redfin are helpful to narrow your search and reach a realtor who can assist you with the entire procedure. Once again, for both rental and own housing, insurance is an essential, and you will get to know more about it through agents.

Connectivity

The advanced digital era drives daily life, especially in the USA. We cannot imagine a day without them and even as resident we can access the electronic health records from any part of the world. Choosing the type of plans for both mobile and Internet can be done at the same time and must be on our checklist too. The few examples of companies are AT&T, T-mobile, Sprint, Verizon, and others. Researching online for reviews always helps. There will be a few places that provide internet/Wi-Fi with accommodation or with a nominal fee.

Transportation

Public Transportation

Modes of public transportation can be by buses, light rails, and subways that can be seen mostly in largely populated metro cities. If you get matched into a rural community program, it is difficult to see such good transportations. The advanced wave of taxis like Uber and Lyft has become available even in the remote places. Still, on average, public transit is deficient in the USA.

Own Transportation

As mentioned above, due to the lack of adequate public transportation, owning a car is not a luxury instead of an essential one. It affords the flexibility to travel around, and parking places are easily usable for residents in every hospital only for a minimal fee. Once again, we need to restate the importance of automobile insurance, which is indispensable. If you chose to get a car, look for the local DMV (Department of Motor Vehicles) where you start working on it.

Food

Arriving from many different countries have different food uses. Globalization is seen in every aspect, especially food secondary to the digital revolution. Decades ago, it was a difficult task to find a specific type of cuisines in the United States. Now there are innumerable resources to find the produce, and net surfing provides you with the best restaurants around the place you live. Being a physician and having knowledge about the food adds up to your patient care by counseling, if they follow a very unhealthy dietary lifestyle.

Conclusion

The USA, land of opportunities and dreams, has much more to explore. In conclusion, we hope the information we provided helps you with all facets of your life in the USA, while you unfold your journey as a resident.

References

1. https://www.ncbi.nlm.nih.gov/pubmed/8709665.
2. Escarce JJ, Kapur K. 10 access to and quality of health care. In: Hispanics and the future of America. Washington, DC: National Academies Press; 2006.
3. https://www.ncbi.nlm.nih.gov/pubmed/9794340.
4. https://www.ncbi.nlm.nih.gov/pubmed/12509547.
5. A Practitioner's Guide to Ethical Decision Making Holly Forester-Miller, Ph.D. Thomas Davis, Ph.D.

Chapter 30
What Should I Pack and Not?

Sorabh Datta

Ready... Get Set... Go!!

From the start of the March month, time seemed to be longer. I thought my watch was slowed down, and the Match Day looked to be far. That waiting period was the most challenging phase of my life. It was like a feeling of helplessness where I felt that I don't have any control over it. Then came the Match Day, I was sitting with my mom chatting about something when I heard the email notification sound DING! Upon unlocking my phone, I saw four missed phone calls, a handful of text messages from friends and an email notification which upon opening read *"Congratulations! You have matched!"* This was probably the most critical email in my USMLE's journey. I was having all the emotions at that moment, from the tears of joy to the flashback of USMLE memories, everything played in that minute like a symphony. Now after been matched in my top choice, WHAT'S NEXT? How should I plan my trip for the next phase of my life (which is the residency)? *What should I pack and not pack?* This chapter will give you the answers to all these essential questions.

For IMGs residing outside the United States of America, moving out of their house to a new place is never an easy thing. As you will be moving to the United States, that too for quite

S. Datta (✉)
Pravara Institute of Medical Sciences, Ahmednagar, India

© Springer Nature Switzerland AG 2020   187
R. Govindarajan et al. (eds.), *International Medical Graduate and the United States Medical Residency Application*,
https://doi.org/10.1007/978-3-030-31045-5_30

a long time, you have to make sure that you have all the necessary stuff with you. Nowadays all kind of groceries, clothing, electronics, etc. is available in the United States, all thanks to the advancement in the global trading system. A person doesn't have to carry everything when leaving for the United States. Obviously, no one can replace the sweets made by your mother, but at the same time, we have to be aware that what all items we can or can't bring to the United States. The US Customs and Border Protection (CBP) regulate all the products imported to the United States, and we have to make sure that we should comply with their regulations. The CBP will give you the Customs Declaration Form 6059B which is for the declaration of goods that have been imported to the United States and failing to do so can result in up to $10,000 in fines and penalties. Below is Table 30.1 showing the acceptable and the unacceptable items as per the latest CBP guidelines:

Moving and packing are the two nightmares we all have to deal with while moving to a new place for our residency. In that excitement and nervousness, we tend to forget packing important stuff, but thanks to an amazing global shipping system, everything is 3–5 days away from you.

Moving

- Make sure that for accommodation, we should take the help of the program coordinator and the residents. Their advice will be far better than any online reviews.
- Now that you have something in your pocket from the residency, you can surely think about the fancy home you were looking for your residency period. But just remember "saving is amazing" and keep a balance between your expenditure and savings.
- For rental properties, the following websites can help:
  - www.apartments.com
  - www.forrent.com
  - www.rentjungle.com
- For buying homes, the following websites can help:
  - www.realtor.com
  - www.trulia.com
  - www.zillow.com

TABLE 30.1 Acceptable and the unacceptable items as per the latest CBP guidelines

Imported items	Permissible	Prohibited
Food	Unopened and commercially packed.	Loose burlap packaging.
Fruits and vegetables	Needed to be clean and must be presented to CBP officer for inspection.	May be prohibited if they contain any insects or diseases.
Animal products and animal by-products	Beef products from the country which are free from Bovine Spongiform Encephalopathy (BSE) and Foot-and-Mouth Disease (FMD).	Fresh, dried or canned meats or meat products is generally not allowed
Medicines	Drugs in their original container along with the prescription.	Narcotics with a high potential for abuse— Rohypnol, GHB, and Fen-Phen

• For packing and moving, the following websites can help:
  – www.moving.com
  – www.movingscam.com
  – www.unpakt.com

Packing

Along with the stress of visa and moving, packing also plays an important role. This chapter will further guide you in packing important stuff.

• Most of the international flights allow us to check in two bags per passenger:
  – *Economy class*: Maximum weight per bag is 50 lbs. (23 kg) with maximum exterior dimensions of 62 inches.
  – *Business/first class*: Maximum weight per bag is 70 lbs. (32 kg) with maximum exterior dimensions of 62 inches.
• Make a checklist of all the important documents:

Identification passport (please check expiration date), driver's license, visa papers, flight tickets and information, certificates (birth, academic, wedding, medical, and vaccination records), ERAS and USMLE documents, documents of the program where you matched, accommodation details, bank and property papers, health/travel insurance policies, loan papers, and list of contacts of people in the United States and back in your home country (in case of emergency).

- Also, make the scanned photocopies of the all the above-mentioned documents and leave at least one copy of each back in your home country.
- Take your credit and debit cards (for ATM withdrawals), and try to carry some cash with you. Also carry smaller denominations (20$, 10$, 5$, 1$).
- Try to pack minimum clothes as you can buy more after you move at your destination. Carry shirts (up to 5), pants (2), one pair of a suit, underwear and socks (5), two pairs of dress shoes, ties or scarf (3), sleepwear/loungewear, a quick-dry towel, sweater/lightweight fleece, and jacket (especially if you are matched at a cold place).
- In electronics, your mobile phone, portable power banks, chargers and batteries, laptop/tablet, USB flash drive, digital camera, and headphones. Make sure they are in your carry-on luggage. Many airlines won't allow checked-in portable power banks, chargers, and batteries.
- Toiletries are something you don't have to worry about as you can go to any nearby superstores like Wal-Mart, Target, etc. Take as little as you can, just for the trip to your destination. Remember the rule *pack less and enjoy more* (make sure to follow the Transportation Security Administration's 3-1-1 rule)
- And don't forget to pack the important things which are near to your heart and soul.

Following Fig. 30.1 will help you in packing your suitcase efficiently.

Remember to pack light to enjoy the sweet freedom of true mobility. Happy travels!

Packing suitcase hacks:
Step 1: Roll all your clothes now it will not look wrinkly.

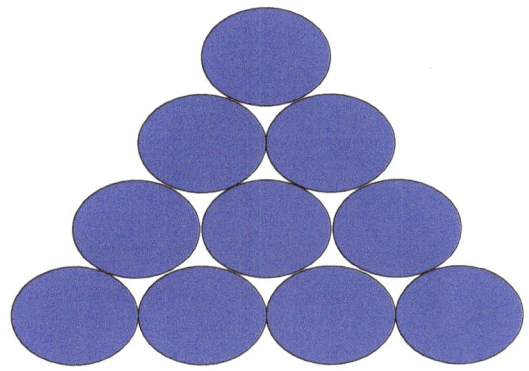

(This is how rolled clothes will look like)

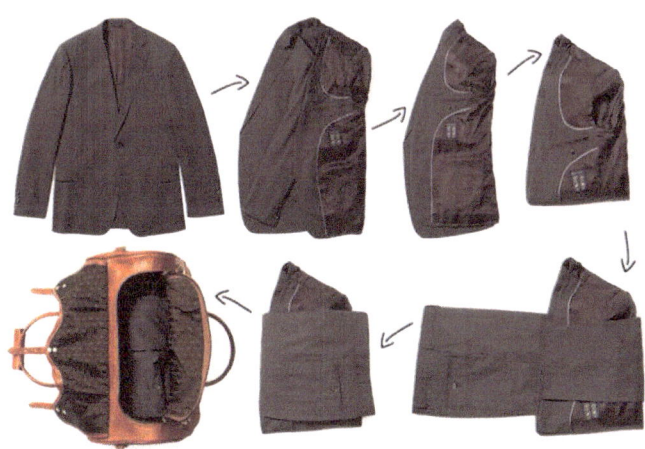

One pair of suit folded along their natural seams.

(Suit folded along their seams)

FIGURE 30.1 A step-by-step illustration of how you can pack in your suitcase

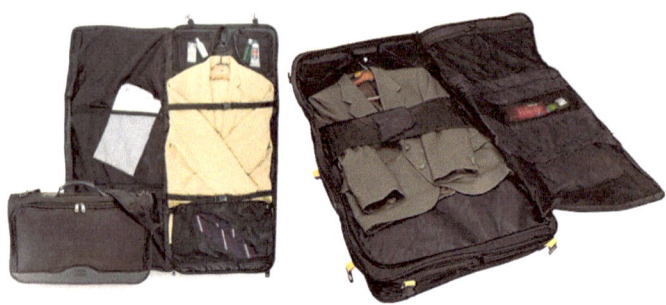

One pair of suit in a carry-on garment bag
(in case when your check-in luggage is misplaced by the airlines)

Step 2: Lay your shoes along the wall of the luggage.

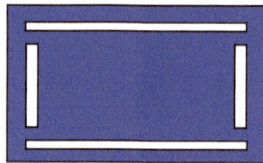

Step 3: Put pants at the bottom

Step 4: Next layer- sweaters and shirts

Step 5: Now put all your rolled clothes (from Step 1). Put rolls tight

Step 6: Cosmetic bag, toiletry bag on the top.

FIGURE 30.1 (continued)

Chapter 31
When Can I Go Back to See My Family?

Sorabh Datta

The love of a family is life's greatest blessing

Family is the single most influence in anyone's life (Fig. 31.1). A family is your parents who are your first teachers, your support and your shelter. A family is your siblings who taught you the importance of sharing; a family is your better half and your children who will motivate you during your residency career. And last but not the least family is your friends who have been with you from your bad times to your good times. All these people are influential in your life.

Residency itself is a challenging period in anyone's life, and most of the residency duration is 3–7 years, it can be longer if fellowship plans are added. For IMGs coming from outside the United States that amount of time away from your loved ones is definitely not easy if not difficult. You will gain new friends and family during the residency period, but the vital question that every IMGs have is when they will go back to see their family again? This chapter will help you in dealing with this important question.

S. Datta (✉)
Pravara Institute of Medical Sciences, Ahmednagar, India

© Springer Nature Switzerland AG 2020
R. Govindarajan et al. (eds.), *International Medical Graduate and the United States Medical Residency Application*,
https://doi.org/10.1007/978-3-030-31045-5_31

193

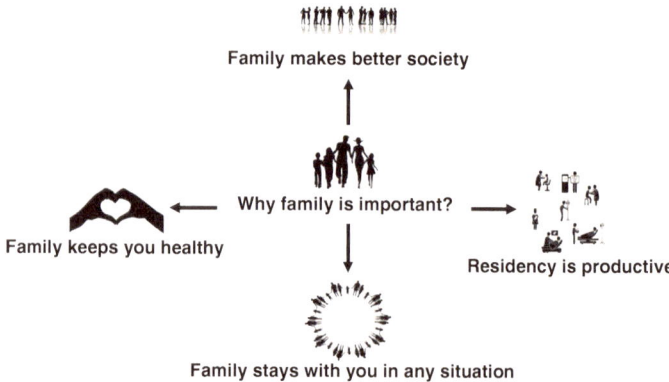

F<small>IGURE</small> 31.1   Illustrates how family can be very important if life

Vacations policies vary from program to program and are limited with 2–3 weeks off in a year, which you can mostly decide to take at once or split it. Residents mostly use this period to go back to see their family members. There are various types of leave system, and we will talk briefly about them.

- *Parental Leave (family leave)*: After the delivery, a resident may have a certain number of days as leave during the postpartum period.
- *Resident Vacation*: 3–4 weeks of leave per academic year.
- *Educational Leave*: Residents can have the educational leave the year they are applying for their fellowships, during poster/abstract/research presentations, during USMLE Step 3 examination.
- *Personal and Discretionary Leave*: In this resident can opt for the leave for reasons like weddings, religious holidays.
- *Sick Leave*: In this, the residents can take off from work due to their health issues and they will get the leave without losing their pay.

- *Jury Duty*: Residents are excused for their jury service and related travel.
- *Military Leave*: Residents are excused from their training program to fulfill their military obligations/service.

Why Visa Is Important for IMGs?

IMGs must obtain an appropriate visa that allows them to get residency training here in the United States (US). The Educational Commission for Foreign Medical Graduates (ECFMG) is authorized by the US government to sponsor the J-1 Visa to the foreign national physicians as "Exchange Visitors" [1].

What Are the Important Regulations That IMGs Have to Follow After Getting the J-1 Visa?

- As per section 212(e) of the Immigration and Nationality Act, as amended, J-1 physicians and their accompanying J-2 dependents should stay in their home country for at least 2 years before being eligible for any changes in their visa status in the USA [2].
- Moonlighting is not allowed.
- ECFMG will sponsor the J-1 visa up to the maximum duration of 7 years.
- J-1 physicians must depart the USA within 30 days of the completion of their training (as per the dates mentioned on their Form DS-2019) [3].
- J-1 physicians should have a valid J-1 visa stamped on their passport while reentering the United States except for the Canadian citizens who do not require stamping while reentering. Instead they can present the endorsed (Exchange Visitor Sponsorship Program) EVSP's DS-2019 Form upon reentry to the USA.

What Are the Essential Documents J-1 Physician and J-2 Dependents Should Carry for International Travel?

- Valid passport.
- Valid J-1 visa (Note: Canadian citizens don't require this).
- DS-2019 Form along with the signature from the ECFMG personal validating the document.
- Get your J-1 visa renewed before reentry to the USA (if it is expired).
- Form I-94 with an arrival-departure record.
- J-1 physicians along with their J-2 dependents should also carry the health and the medical insurance records while traveling and upon reentry the USA.
- Travel document is a special document which should be obtained from the International Office of your hospital which you should carry along with your valid DS and should be presented during immigration. Do not forget to apply for travel document before planning to travel outside the USA. Typically it is valid for 1 year (as long the DS is) and hence has to be obtained every year.

What to Expect When Reentering the USA?

- A CBP officer will inspect your documents [4].
- After inspection of all the required documents, CBP officer will issue the Form I-94.
- I-94 Form should contain the latest dates along with the duration of the status for the J-1 visa. If any error or the abovementioned thing is not present on the I-94 Form, then get it corrected from the CBP officer [5].

Important Links

1. US Department of State Exchange Visitor Program
2. US Citizenship and Immigration Services

3. US Department of Homeland Security
4. US Bureau of Consular Affairs' International Travel site
5. US embassy/consulate

Tips for Managing Your Vacation During the Residency

- Always try to split your vacation holidays. For example, if you have 4 weeks of leave in a year, try to split it in 1 week or 2 weeks instead of using the whole 4 weeks.
- You can be productive in the vacation by devoting some time for your research and making some good connections with the faculty members.
- You can also use this time to re-evaluate yourself for your future fellowship plans. You can dedicate 1 week for all this.
- Remember the more hard work you will put into your residency, the more you will get out of your residency.

Last but not least, enjoy your vacation to the fullest with your family, as family is the source of your existence and your support.

References

1. Exchange Visitor Sponsorship Program (EVSP). www.ecfmg.org/evsp/evsprfgd.pdf. Accessed 23 Dec 2018.
2. § 41.62 Exchange visitors|USCIS. https://www.uscis.gov/ilink/docView/22CFR/HTML/22CFR/0-0-0-1/0-0-0-500/0-0-0-1363.html. Accessed 23 Dec 2018.
3. About DS-2019|Participants|J-1 Visa. https://j1visa.state.gov/participants/how-to-apply/about-ds-2019/. Accessed 23 Dec 2018.
4. Automatic Revalidation. https://travel.state.gov/content/travel/en/us-visas/visa-information-resources/visa-expiration-date/auto-revalidate.html. Accessed 23 Dec 2018.
5. ECFMG|EVSP: Travel. https://www.ecfmg.org/evsp/applicants-current-travel.html. Accessed 23 Dec 2018.

Timeline at a Glance

TIMELINE AT A GLANCE...

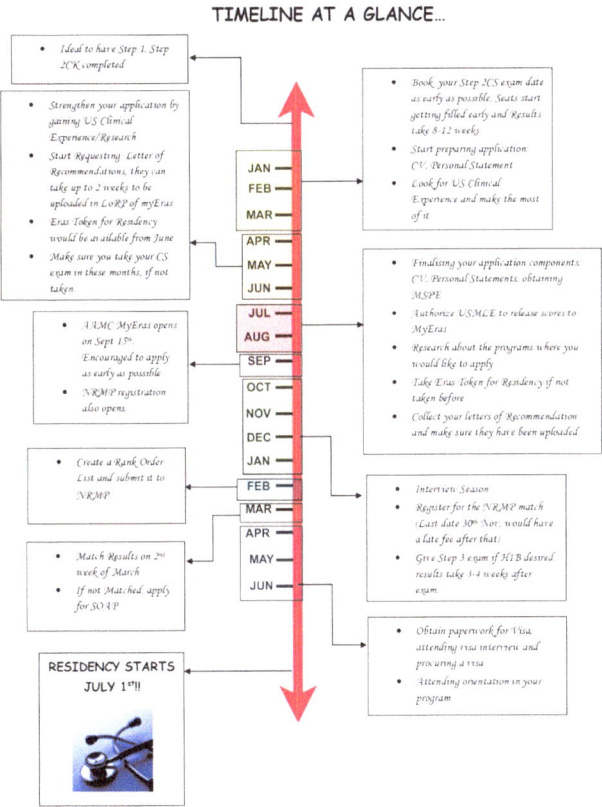

- Ideal to have Step 1, Step 2CK completed

- Strengthen your application by gaining US Clinical Experience/Research
- Start Requesting Letter of Recommendations; they can take up to 2 weeks to be uploaded in LoRP of myEras
- Eras Token for Residency would be available from June
- Make sure you take your CS exam in these months, if not taken

- AAMC MyEras opens on Sept 15th. Encouraged to apply as early as possible
- NRMP registration also opens

- Create a Rank Order List and submit it to NRMP

- Match Results on 2nd week of March
- If not Matched, apply for SOAP

RESIDENCY STARTS JULY 1st!!

JAN
FEB
MAR
APR
MAY
JUN
JUL
AUG
SEP
OCT
NOV
DEC
JAN
FEB
MAR
APR
MAY
JUN

- Book your Step 2CS exam date as early as possible. Seats start getting filled early and Results take 8-12 weeks
- Start preparing application CV, Personal Statement
- Look for US Clinical Experience and make the most of it

- Finalising your application components. CV, Personal Statements, obtaining MSPE
- Authorize USMLE to release scores to MyEras
- Research about the programs where you would like to apply
- Take Eras Token for Residency if not taken before
- Collect your letters of Recommendation and make sure they have been uploaded

- Interview Season
- Register for the NRMP match (Last date 30th Nov. would have a late fee after that)
- Give Step 3 exam if H1B desired results take 3-4 weeks after exam

- Obtain paperwork for Visa, attending visa interview and procuring a visa
- Attending orientation in your program

© Springer Nature Switzerland AG 2020   199
R. Govindarajan et al. (eds.), *International Medical Graduate and the United States Medical Residency Application*,
https://doi.org/10.1007/978-3-030-31045-5

Index

© Springer Nature Switzerland AG 2020
R. Govindarajan et al. (eds.), *International Medical Graduate and the United States Medical Residency Application*,
https://doi.org/10.1007/978-3-030-31045-5